Reading, Writing and Speech Problems in Children
───────────

Reading, Writing and Speech Problems in Children

A Presentation of Certain Types of Disorders in the Development of the Language Faculty

BY SAMUEL TORREY ORTON, M.D.
*Former Professor of Neurology and Neuropathology
Columbia University*

W. W. NORTON & COMPANY, INC.
NEW YORK

Copyright, 1937, by
W. W. NORTON & COMPANY, INC.
COPYRIGHT RENEWED, 1964, BY JUNE L. ORTON

Number four in the Thomas William Salmon
Memorial Lecture Series

ISBN 0 393 1107 0 (Paperback edition)
ISBN 0 393 01032 5 (Cloth edition)
PRINTED IN THE UNITED STATES OF AMERICA
234567890

TO

J. L. O.

Contents

FOREWORD 11

INTRODUCTION 13

I. LANGUAGE LOSSES IN THE ADULT AS THE KEY TO THE DEVELOPMENTAL DISORDERS IN CHILDREN 21
    UNILATERAL CEREBRAL DOMINANCE 27
    THE APHASIAS 35
        1. *Alexia (Word Blindness)* 37
        2. *Auditory Aphasia (Word Deafness)* 39
        3. *Motor Agraphia* 44
        4. *Motor Aphasia* 45
        5. *Apraxia* 47
    LATERALITY (HANDEDNESS, EYEDNESS, ETC.) 48
    STUDIES IN LATERALITY 51
    MOTOR INTEGRADING 61

II. CERTAIN DISORDERS IN THE DEVELOPMENT OF LANGUAGE IN CHILDREN 68
    DESCRIPTION OF SYNDROMES 69

Contents

1. *Developmental Alexia (The Reading Disability)* 69
2. *Developmental Agraphia (Special Writing Disability)* 99
3. *Developmental Word Deafness* 111
4. *Developmental Motor Aphasia (Motor Speech Delay)* 118
5. *Developmental Apraxia (Abnormal Clumsiness)* 120
6. *Stuttering in Childhood* 122
7. *Combined or Mixed Syndromes* 126

HEREDITARY FACTORS 127

EMOTIONAL REACTIONS AND BEHAVIOR PATTERNS 131

III. INTERPRETATION AND TREATMENT OF CERTAIN DISORDERS OF LANGUAGE IN CHILDREN 142

INTERPRETATION 144

TREATMENT 156

1. *Developmental Alexia* 158
2. *Developmental Agraphia* 179
3. *Developmental Word Deafness* 185
4. *Developmental Motor Aphasia* 187
5. *Developmental Apraxia* 190
6. *Stuttering in Childhood* 194

CONCLUSION 200

GLOSSARY 201

INDEX 215

List of Illustrations

1. *A map of the human brain showing its lobes*   32
2. *A map of the visual areas in the brain*   33
3. *A map of the critical language areas of the brain*   40
4. *Educational profile of an eight-year-old boy with a reading disability*   75
5. *Educational profile of a ten-year-old girl with a reading disability*   75
6. *Educational profile of a fourteen-year-old girl with a reading disability*   76
7. *Confusion between* b *and* d *and* p *and* q *in the writing of an eight-year-old boy*   81
8. *Confusion in orientation of letters and direction of writing from the work of a ten-year-old girl*   81
9. *Educational profile of a case of special disability in spelling*   86
10. *Unintelligible composition produced by a sixteen-year-old boy with a reading disability*   88
11. *A simpler composition by the same boy whose work is shown in Figure 10*   88

List of Illustrations

12. *Letter perfect copy by the same boy who produced Figures 10 and 11*   89
13. *Educational profile of a case of special writing disability*   100
14. *Effect of retraining the writing of a shifted left-handed boy of fifteen*   102
15. *Effect of retraining the writing in a case of masked left-handedness*   103
16. *Spontaneous mirror-writing by a left-handed boy*   104
17. *Good mirror-writing skill with poor ability to write in the ordinary direction*   106
18. *Good mirror-writing in a case of special writing disability*   108
19. *Skillful writing in either direction with either hand*   109
20. *Comparison of writing while blindfolded and while watching the paper*   110
21. *Audiogram in a case of high frequency deafness*   115
22. *Nine family charts showing the incidence of left-handedness and language disorders*   129
23. *Cross-section of spinal cord showing antitropism of motor cell groups*   154
24. *Left- and right-handed positions for writing*   182

Foreword

THE commanding position which Dr. Thomas W. Salmon made for himself in American psychiatry both during the war and in the years that followed in his professorship at Columbia imposes a responsibility of no mean magnitude on the recipient of the lectureship created in his honor and in his memory. Nor is this obligation in any way lessened by the outstanding place occupied by those who have given the first three of these memorial lectures.

In the present volume the writer offers a necessarily condensed summary of the findings of a ten-year period of intensive study of some disorders in the acquisition of the language faculty encountered by certain children, as interpreted from a much longer period of interest and study from the literature, in the clinic, at the autopsy table and in the laboratory, of cerebral localization and of the aphasias. The work with children was begun as an outgrowth of an experiment with a mobile Mental Hygiene Unit organized and sent into the field under the writer's direction by the Iowa State Psychopathic Hospital in 1925, and was extended there for a time under a generous grant from the Rockefeller Foundation. From 1930 to 1936 it was continued as the Language Research Project of the New York Neurological Institute, again with aid, during the lean years, from the Rockefeller Foundation.

These last six years of observation and experiment have broadened our experience with diagnostic methods, have served to control the efficacy of training techniques, and have extended therapeutic aid to several hundred children suffering from language delays and disorders. An epitome of the yield of the whole ten-year period is here presented for the first time.

Since any disorder in the normal acquisition of spoken or written language serves as a severe hindrance to academic advancement and often also lies at the root of serious emotional disturbances, the studies here recorded may prove of interest to teachers and parents as well as to physicians, and therefore this presentation has been simplified in so far as its content would permit. The inclusion of some technical words has, however, seemed unavoidable, and for this reason a brief glossary of such words has been appended.

Introduction

MAN'S dominant position in the animal world rests largely if not entirely on his possession of two facilities:—first, his ability to make use of sounds, markings and gestures for the purpose of communicating with others of his kind and as a background for his own ideation and, second, the very high degree of skill which he has developed in the use of his hands since they were freed from the duties of support and locomotion by the abandonment of the arboreal habit and adoption of the erect posture.

In most of the simpler functions of the nervous system man seems to be definitely inferior to some one or another of his animal competitors. Mention need only be made here of the superiority of most mammals in the sense of smell, of the strikingly greater acuity of vision possessed by the soaring birds of prey by virtue of their second macula, of the exquisite vibratory sense of many fish, and of the fact that certain insects—notably the honeybee—are capable of responding to light waves in the ultra-violet which are well beyond the range of human vision. It is therefore of arresting interest to note that in the two faculties whence man's superiority derives—speech and manual dexterity—a highly novel physiological pattern has been evolved in the brain whereby the functional control of these faculties is restricted sharply to one of the two cerebral hemispheres—a plan of activity in sharp contrast to that existing in the lower functional units of the central nervous system where exact bilateral symmetry is the rule.

That the higher animals other than man possess a means of communicating with each other is obvious, but the content of such communication is limited strictly to the transfer from one to another of the feeling tone of the moment. Considerable confusion has arisen in discussions of animal "language" because of failure clearly to recognize this limitation. Thus the emotional state of the animal is expressed in the sounds which it emits or the bodily postures which it exhibits and one who is well acquainted with his dog, for example, can tell by either the bark or the postures whether it be excited or angry or forlorn.

Nor has man lost this facility of communicating feeling tones. Indeed in early infancy this "animal language" is his only equipment and almost from the beginning the baby shows a high degree of the capacity to react in harmony to the emotional state of his mother or his nurse and is able also to give expression to many types of his own feelings so accurately that the experienced mother can very often tell from the sound of the child's cry alone whether he be hungry or frightened or in pain. Volume, pitch, and timbre of the voice, the occurrence of vibrato and a wide range of associated movements of the face and body all play their part in this emotional expression which is never entirely lost from human speech, although the extent to which it is exhibited varies markedly with the individual, with race, and with training. As might be expected from its long phylogenetic ancestry this form of expression which depicts the feelings has become very deeply rooted in the nervous system and may today be characterized as subserved by an instinctive or reflex mechanism which requires no training. Cannon and his co-workers have demonstrated that, in the cat, centers which are capable of controlling emotional expression are to be found in the thalamic region which is a part of the nervous system far older phylogenetically than is the true brain. Emotional expression is well developed in earliest infancy while the cortex is still extremely immature, as well as in cases of very marked defect in the development of the brain. Indeed certain rare cases of deformity in which a child is born without any brain whatsoever (anencephalic monsters) have been able to cry and to exhibit the appropriate accompanying facial expression. Conversely, emotional expression is usually retained late in the dementias and is often to be seen preserved in full vigor in extensive aphasic syndromes.

In man, however, in contrast to all other animals, another form of communication has evolved and it is this which primarily interests us here. This is symbolic language, in which a sign or a series of sounds has come to serve as a substitute for an object or a concept and can thus be used as a means of transferring ideas rather than mere feeling tone to a second individual. As mentioned above, that fraction of our language which deals with emotional expression is instinctive and requires no instruction, but it is obvious that if symbolic language is to carry meaning between two individuals they must both learn to associate the same symbol with the same object or idea, and thus it is that we find this form of language always dependent upon training. The acquisition of verbal language understanding and response by the normal child is such a gradual and effortless process that it is sometimes difficult to appreciate that this is a result of specific teaching until we remember that the child learns the language, be it English, French or German, to which he is exposed, while his emotional expressions are so independent of teaching as to be universally understandable.

Communication of meaning may be accomplished by spoken sounds, by written or printed characters, or by symbolic gestures, and thus we may delineate the language faculty as the capacity to understand the spoken word and to reproduce it verbally, the capacity to understand the written word and to reproduce it, and, less commonly used, the ability to understand and to reproduce gestures which carry specific meaning as in the sign language.

As already mentioned, that part of the language faculty which deals with the emotional moment probably has a very long phylogenetic history extending well back into the animal series. As measured by this, symbolic language is without doubt a relatively recent acquisition although it still is of an age to command respect. We know nothing with security about the time of development of speech or of sign language, but the earliest known fossil skulls of man give evidence of a brain development which would have been sufficient for such needs and man as far back as we can trace him already knew how to fashion crude weapons, so we may assume that the skills needed for symbolic gestures were already at hand and Sir Richard Paget has offered an interesting thesis that the sign language was

Introduction 17

the first form of symbolic language to be developed and that spoken language was largely an outgrowth therefrom. Studies of the brain case in fossil man show not only that his brain was greatly enlarged in size over that of the anthropoids but that this expansion had taken place in the frontal and parietal lobes which include all the critical areas which subserve both spoken and written language in modern man. The exact age of these examples of fossil man cannot of course be determined, but they probably extend back at least a half a million years. Sign language was extensively used by the American Indian for inter-communication between tribes who had a large number of different dialects, but in most races which have developed a spoken language it has undergone degeneration almost to the vanishing point if, as Paget believes, it was the origin of the spoken form. In contrast to the probable great age of spoken language, and possibly also of sign language as well, written language is probably only a few thousand years old.

The development of speech in the child is generally believed to go through several stages. The first of these is the lal or babbling period during which the infant produces many vowel sounds usually linked with a consonant and often with the same consonant repeated after the vowel. Labial consonants predominate and pure linguals are less frequent. The second stage is that of echolalia or echo speech which is characterized by an immediate repetition of words heard but without any understanding of their meaning and without the ability to reproduce them except as an echo. Usually the period in which the echo speech is used exclusively by the child is quite short and any consider-

18   Introduction

able elongation of this period is apt to be indicative of a delay in the maturation of the higher form of speech although a minor degree of echoing may persist for some time along with the beginnings of real speech. Clearly this ability to echo even quite complex word sounds is still a very lowly form of integration of the motor speech mechanism with the auditory centers since no association is built with meaning. Its interest for us lies in the fact that it is often stated that comprehension of the word, that is lalognosis, precedes its reproduction. Obviously this is not true of echolalia as quite a range of complicated motor patterns are involved in the echo process long before any recognition of their symbolic meaning occurs. This question as to whether the understanding of words precedes the development of speech need not detain us here, however, as it is quite evident that children follow no general rule in this regard since we see in childhood—and indeed in adult life also—individuals with poor word memory and paucity both of understanding and of speech, others with good understanding but poor expression, and finally those with a quick ear for words and a facile tongue for their repetition but with very little comprehension. In some children the understanding of the spoken word clearly precedes the development of their speech; in others the reverse is apparently true.

As we have stated, the infant's instinctive or reflex capacity to communicate its emotional states is present from the beginning of its independent life but gradually there is evolved an association of certain word sounds with objects of the environment and as this symbolic speech increases, the child's dependence on emo-

Introduction 19

tional expression is reciprocally reduced. The character and efficiency of the training methods employed at this point are a cardinal factor in the degree with which the emotional expression will be inhibited, but other variables also enter here. Thus the child who is delayed in his development of verbal symbolism will continue to· use, over a longer period and to a greater extent, his emotional expression and naturally demands and receives a greater share of maternal protection than he would were he better able to understand commands and express his desires. Many such obvious psychological factors—especially those affecting emotional maturation—as well as many environmental influences play an important role in the development of language, but even after making abundant allowance for all such variations it is apparent to the critical observer that there are striking inherent or constitutional differences in certain children, apart from those of general intelligence, which markedly influence their acquisition of the language function, and it is toward the better understanding of these differences and of their most satisfactory treatment that the studies which are reported in this volume were directed.

We are all familiar with the progress from the echo period to the use, first, of nouns, then verbs, and later sentences, and the gradual lengthening of the sequences of words and phrases which characterize development at this period. In the average child this increasing familiarity with the spoken word both for understanding and response forms the only development in his language function during the first six years of his life. By the time he has reached school age it has been estimated that the normal child has an understanding vocabulary of several thousand words. This forms the foundation on which he must begin, at the age of six or thereabouts, to erect an entirely new form of language—reading and writing—if he is to take his place in the literate world. In the occasional very precocious child, reading and writing can be taught much before the age of six, but taking our school population at large, attempts at teaching graphic language before this age are unprofitable and it seems probable that it is this fact which has determined the age of six for an introduction to formal academic training. It may therefore be pertinent to inquire whether the cortices of the angular gyrus region have reached a sufficient anatomical or physiological maturity before this period to make reading and writing practicable. If this should prove to be the explanation it would constitute an interesting ontogenetic parallel with the relative age of spoken and written languages.

Chapter One

LANGUAGE LOSSES IN THE ADULT AS THE KEY TO THE DEVELOPMENTAL DISORDERS IN CHILDREN

MOST of our knowledge of the cerebral physiology of the language faculty is derived from studies of the symptoms which follow injury or disease of the brain in the adult. Thus the extent and character of a disturbance in speech, in reading or in writing which follows damage to the brain may be studied and after the patient's death the brain may be removed and carefully dissected to determine just what parts of it have suffered injury. Such an approach of necessity limits our investigations to the slow accretion of facts gathered by many investigators and over a long period of time and is obviously much less precise than the direct experimental attack which is possible in many fields of medicine. Moreover, it is beset with many inherent difficulties. Neither injury nor disease is apt to be limited by anatomical boundaries, and in both the damage to the brain is very prone to overlap two or more areas of the brain which have quite different functions and hence to lead to confusion in interpretation. One of the commonest causes of such partial brain destruction is the blocking of an artery with consequent starvation and death of the nerve cells and fibers in the area which it fed, and since there are few arteries of any considerable size in the brain which do not serve more than one functional brain area, the effect of such vascular disease is usually complex. Moreover, the majority of the vascular accidents which lead to blocking of an artery are the result of arteriosclerosis which is a diffuse process involving many arteries so that more than one area of damage is very often found in such cases. Again, arteriosclerosis of the brain vessels is a slowly progressive disease and new areas of destruction and new resultant symptoms may occur and interfere seriously with interpretation unless the studies of the patient's speech have been made shortly before his death.

A second common cause of brain damage is by the growth of a brain tumor, and here the results are apt to be even more confusing because the damage is produced in part at least through the pressure exerted by the growing tumor, and such pressure effects may be transferred to other parts of the brain than those where the tumor is growing and hence give rise to misleading or confusing symptoms. Direct injuries of the brain through wounds which break or penetrate the skull are sometimes circumscribed but not uncommonly they also spread over areas of the brain which have two or more functions. Not infrequently we see transient disturbances in speech or reading occurring in patients with high blood pressure which are probably due to a spasm of a small artery. These attacks which are commonly described as a threatened stroke are, in the writer's experience, very apt to be highly selective in the sense that they disturb only one fraction of the language faculty but they do not as a rule result in permanent damage to the brain cells so that the exact locus of the brain areas involved cannot be established

Problems in Children

with certainty if an autopsy should be performed later. In recent years, as brain surgery has advanced, operations for the excision of malignant brain tumors have often included removal of large parts of brain substance adjacent to the tumor and careful studies of the symptoms shown by these patients after operation are opening a new avenue of information. Unfortunately here again it is often very difficult to be sure of just how much of the brain substance has been removed, since a tumor—particularly a slowly growing one—may often cause marked pressure displacement of brain substance without interfering seriously with its function and it is therefore at times impossible to determine whether a given area has been removed or had been crowded aside before the operation.

Animal experiments are of no value in this problem since even the highest of the apes lack the very functions and to a large extent the brain areas in which we are interested and, moreover, it is a well established fact that the physiological activities of the brain of one phylum cannot be used for interpretation of those of another. Many observations point to the fact that there is a progressive concentration of functional control in the true brain as the animal scale is ascended and that some functions which in man are exclusively resident in the brain cortex, in some of the animals are partly at least governed by lower nerve centers. In man's brain, for example, the optic thalami—two large collections of nerve cells lying at the base of the true brain—have been reduced as far as vision is concerned to nerve relay stations between the eyes and the cortex, and will not serve for vision, whereas in the dog—an animal relatively high in the scale—experiments have been recorded indicating that the thalami will serve to discriminate between light and dark, and in birds and reptiles almost all of vision is controlled by these structures and very little by the brain cortex. A comparable situation is to be seen in control of motion. In man, destruction of the brain cortex of the motor area causes a complete and permanent paralysis of voluntary movement of the corresponding muscles; in the anthropoids a minor amount of recovery of voluntary motion takes place after destruction of the motor cortex, while in the lower monkeys recovery after such destruction is practically complete. Failure to understand that the brain of man is, except in name, not the same functional organ as that of the lower animals has led to much loose thinking and many futile attempts to discuss human brain physiology on the basis of findings in the white rat or other experimental animal.

Still another obstacle to the study of the cerebral physiology of language arises from the fact that in the normal adult the various functions which make up the language faculty—speaking, reading, writing, etc.—are so closely interlinked both in learning and by usage that any interference with one seems prone to cause disturbance of others. Thus, loss of the capacity to read, for example, without some degradation of speech is exceedingly rare. It is probable that a large individual variation enters here also and that those who have been extensive readers and have stocked their vocabulary largely through this route would show a different degree of speech disorder resulting from a loss of reading than would those who have learned words chiefly by ear. Such factors cannot at present be evaluated but the element of a common approach to words through both vision and hearing would not appear, of course, in the congenitally deaf or congenitally blind and studies of disturbances in symbolization comparable to the aphasias in such cases should prove progressively informative.

A close co-operation between the clinic and the laboratory is essential to progress here. All too often reports are to be found in the literature of cases excellently studied from the clinical standpoint but with exceedingly inadequate anatomical reports, and again we see extensive anatomical studies carried out on cases with a very meager clinical background. Both approaches are arduous and time-consuming and rarely indeed does the busy practicing clinician have the time and opportunity to study these cases with the care that must be given them if they are to be made to give their greatest yield, and this applies with almost equal force to the laboratory investigations where really thorough studies of one case from the localizing standpoint require a major time allotment both by technicians and microscopist. The greatest promise for progress in this complex field of research would seem to rest in especially created and endowed institutes for brain study such as are already to be found in several European centers.

Because of difficulties of investigation such as those mentioned above, the problem of disorders in the language function in the adult is far from being a completed study, but an enormous amount of medical literature has nevertheless accrued during the last seventy-five years and from this and from the writer's own experience in the clinic and laboratory we may select some facts which are believed to be of importance in understanding the obstacles which are encountered by certain children in gaining a normal mastery of spoken and written language. The first of these is that the locus of an area of brain destruction is of much greater import in determining a language disorder than is the amount of brain tissue destroyed. Thus a very small area of damage in the angular gyrus region may result in a complete loss of the ability to read and write and a marked disturbance in speech as well, while a much greater destruction of tissue in, for example, the frontal region of the brain may give no demonstrable disorder in language. Moreover, when we consider certain critical loci there is no direct relationship between the amount of tissue destroyed and the gravity of the symptoms, as a small lesion in the angular gyrus may give as widespread a language disorder as that which follows one twice its size. Clearly this does not harmonize with the older views of strict cerebral localization of functions, which held that the angular gyrus and its neighboring brain convolutions serve as the storehouse for the visual memory of words. The discrepancy sometimes found here between the small volume of tissue destruction and the extensive loss of function points clearly to the conclusion that we are dealing with a disturbance of cerebral physiology rather than a destruction of areas of registration. Again these facts are clearly out of harmony with Lashley's unfortunate misinterpretation of his earlier experimental material which led him to advance the thesis that the volume of brain tissue destroyed is of more significance than the area involved.

Problems in Children

UNILATERAL CEREBRAL DOMINANCE

A second interesting fact and one which seems to be of major meaning to us in understanding the language disorders of children is that one side of the brain is all important in the language process and the other side either useless or unused. So striking is this that we know that a very small area of destruction in an appropriate area of the controlling or dominant hemisphere of the brain will give rise to extensive loss in speech or reading while an equal area of destruction in exactly the same part of the non-dominant or subjugate hemisphere will be followed by no language disorder whatsoever and indeed will often give no recognizable symptoms. This concentration of the whole control of speech, reading and writing in one half of the brain bears an intimate relation to the development of unilateral manual skill in the individual and is the unique physiological pattern mentioned earlier in this volume as the special attribute of those faculties which have done most to give man his commanding position in the animal world. Many of the higher animals show traces of a preferential use of one side of the body. For example, a dog may consistently use the same paw for scratching at a door or a cat may always choose the same paw in reaching through the bars of its cage for food and a race horse when starting to run will quite consistently lead with the same foot. In all of these examples, however, the responses are so simple that the contra-lateral pattern may easily be substituted and indeed often is if the conditions preceding the act be slightly altered. It would be interesting to know whether any differential effect of right- or left-sided brain lesions could be demonstrated on the much more complicated behavior patterns which could be taught to the higher primates, but so far as the writer is aware no such experiments have been recorded and the weight of current evidence is that the animals below man do not exhibit that unilateral cerebral dominance which forms the hallmark of the language faculty.

In considering this striking fact of the functional supremacy of one brain hemisphere, however, it is essential that we bear in mind not only that it is clearly demonstrable only in man but that even in man it is only in the language faculty and the more intricate manual skills that this specialization is to be found and that, for many of the simpler activities of the brain, the relation of the two hemispheres to each other, while a variable one, is quite different from that underlying speech, reading and writing. Thus the two hemispheres operate quite independently of each other in the control of motion so that damage to the brain cortex of the motor area will regularly give rise to a paralysis of voluntary motion on the opposite side of the body only and destruction of similar areas of both hemispheres would be necessary to completely destroy this function. This is also true of that part of the sensations of pain, touch, temperature and kinaesthesis which reaches the brain cortex and which informs us as to the place of origin on the body of these sensations. In vision the situation is somewhat complex due to the fact that the human eye is equipped with two seeing mechanisms—one for quick scanning vision of a broad field and one for more accurate intake of detail in a much narrower range. The first of these—the peripheral retinal field—is organized like the motor centers as a crossed but independent mechanism so that damage in one hemisphere results in a loss of vision on the opposite side and the patient can no longer see "out of the corner of his eye" in that direction. This is the condition known technically as hemianopsia. In the second visual apparatus—central or macular vision—which gives us the finer detail of things seen and most of our ability to distinguish colors, the two hemispheres seem to work as a unit so that the stimuli received by either eye are fused into a single impression as shown by Sherrington's classical flicker experiments with binocular vision. In the matter of hearing, our information is not quite so precise as it is in vision, but the general opinion is that here, as in central vision, either of the two hemispheres may serve interchangeably with each other. When those parts of the brain cortex which serve as the terminus of nerve paths from the eyes and ears—the so-called arrival platforms—have been destroyed in both hemispheres of the brain, we encounter the conditions known as cortical blindness and cortical deafness, respectively, in which no conscious vision or audition is possible although the eyes and ears are normal.

These lowest anatomical centers, as so far described, are however only the first step in the brain's use of visual and auditory data, and studies of cases with differently placed brain injuries show us that it is possible for a patient to see and hear and yet to be unable to understand the meaning of objects seen or sounds heard. These conditions are those which are called visual and auditory agnosia and the patients are said to be suffering from mind blindness or mind deafness.

The capacity to comprehend the meaning or purpose of objects seen and to understand the various sounds of the environment is usually retained, however, in patients who have lost the capacity to read or to understand the spoken word, and thus we see that there are three steps or levels in the degree of physiological complexity with which the brain makes use of incoming data represented in vision by, respectively, 1st, cortical blindness—in which there is no conscious vision; 2nd, mind blindness—in which the patient can see so that he does not collide with things in moving about but is quite unable to recall the purpose or use of the objects seen; and 3rd, word blindness—in which there is no loss of vision or of the capacity to recognize and interpret objects, pictures, etc., but in which the printed word no longer brings its meaning. The comparable conditions in the field of hearing are cortical deafness, mind deafness and word deafness. Destruction of the appropriate cortex area in *both hemispheres* is necessary before cortical blindness or cortical deafness occurs, and while there is some difference of opinion among investigators here, the majority of students of this problem believe that bilateral destruction is necessary at the second level also before mind blindness and mind deafness result; but all neurologists are agreed that a lesion in one brain hemisphere—providing it be the dominant—is sufficient to cause the disorders of spoken and written language.

Studies of the comparative anatomy of the brain have demonstrated that the striking enlargement which has taken place in man's brain when compared to that of the highest animals is not merely a general increase in total brain volume but is a disproportionate expansion of the third level type of cortex in which are to be found those areas whose integrity is essential for the proper functioning of the language faculty. In the brain of the monkey, the cortex devoted to the first level of vision covers a much larger relative area than it does in the human brain and the cortices of the second and third level are comparatively restricted. Figure 1 is a conventionalized drawing of the two sides of the left hemisphere of a human brain showing the major anatomical subdivisions or lobes. The occipital lobe serves vision exclusively. The temporal lobe is largely auditory although some parts of it probably subserve smell as well. The parietal lobe serves for the reception, registration and elaboration of the senses of touch, pain and temperature and of muscle, tendon and joint sense (kinaesthesis). The functions of the frontal lobe are not completely understood but it contains all of the mechanisms for the elaboration and control of voluntary movements. Certain higher mental attributes have been assigned to this region by various authors but as a whole it may be loosely considered as primarily the executive division of the brain. The limbic lobe has to do with smell and taste and possibly certain of the sensations arising within the body. The parts of the human brain which have undergone the greatest relative expansion as compared to that of the highest primates are the frontal lobe and that area in which the parietal, occipital and temporal lobes meet.

While the separation of the sensory functions into three stages or levels of elaboration, as given above, rests primarily on the study of the symptoms resulting from brain disease or injury, it also receives support

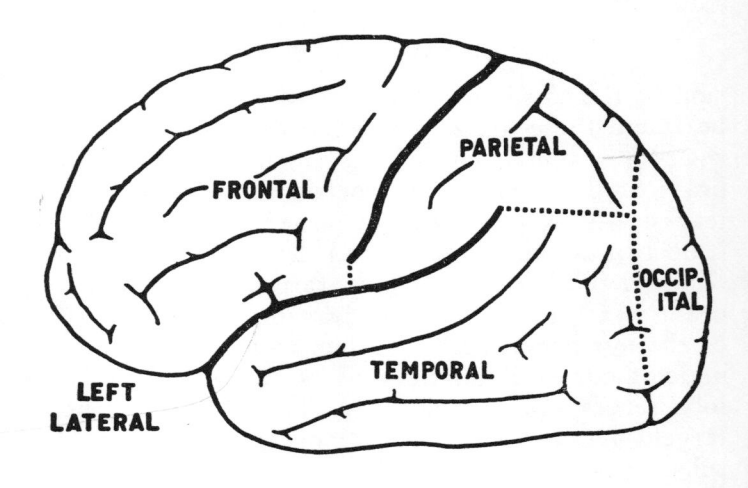

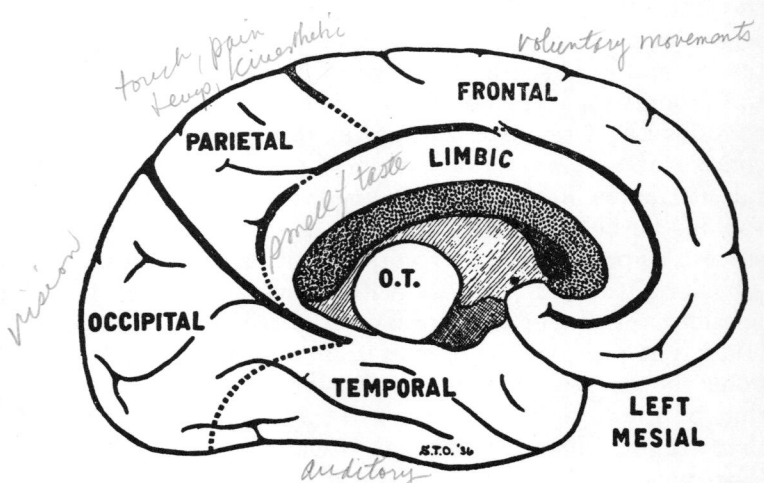

FIGURE 1. *A conventionalized map of the outer (lateral) and inner (mesial) surfaces of the left hemisphere of the human brain showing the location of its major subdivisions or lobes.*

from microscopic studies of the brain cortex, which reveal differences in the size, number and arrangement of the nerve cells and fibers by which the brain areas subserving these various steps can be distinguished

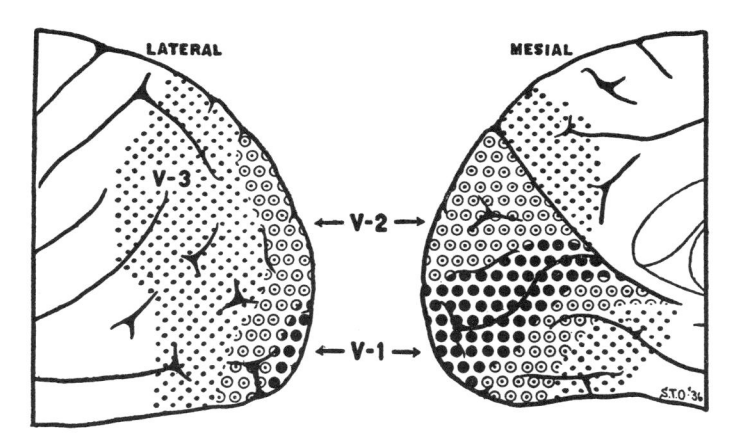

FIGURE 2. *An outline map of the lateral and mesial surfaces of the occipital region of the left hemisphere of a human brain showing the distribution of the three chief types of visual cortex.*

from one another, or to express this in another way, the brain shows structural as well as functional differentiation of these three levels. Figure 2 shows the distribution of the three types of cortex from the structural standpoint which are to be found in the occipital pole or visual area of the brain. The first area—V-1—is known as the area striata because of the presence of a white band of nerve fibers which is so prominent that the confines of this type of cortex can be readily determined by the naked eye. Surrounding this is the "common occipital" cortex—V-2—which grades off with less sharp demarcation into the third or parieto-occipital type—V-3.

Another striking confirmation of the existence of the three steps in brain function comes from studies of maturation or ripening of the brain cortex. In the embryo and infant, before a given brain area has matured, the nerve fibers lack the fat-like sheath or insulation which is later deposited around them. This fatty sheath is called myelin and the ripening process is spoken of as myelinization of the fibers. The myelin sheaths can be readily stained by appropriate methods and thus the progress of the ripening process can be followed by studies of a series of brains from embryos, stillborn children, and infants. Flechsig applied this method and found that maturation proceeds in three distinct waves covering, in separate stages, those areas of the brain cortex whose destruction leads to the three syndromes of cortical blindness, mind blindness and word blindness and the comparable conditions in audition. Flechsig demonstrated that at the time of birth only the "arrival platforms" or first level cortices have received their myelin, that a second period of myelinization follows during the first two or three months after birth which results in the ripening of a second zone of cortex lying near by each arrival platform and that only during the final or third wave does maturation occur in the areas of the third level.

I have emphasized this dissection of the cerebral functions into steps because it offers us some understanding of how a selective loss of reading, for example, in the adult or a selective retardation in learning to read in a child may occur with full visual competence in other regards and thus focuses our attention on the specific and peculiar physiological pattern by which reading and the other language functions are governed.

THE APHASIAS

The term aphasia is one which has undergone considerable change in its scope, and hence a brief outline of its various meanings may be of value to the reader. Unfortunately, the lay press has very widely confused it with amnesia, meaning loss of memory—a very different sort of condition and, of course, an indefensible error. Even in the medical literature, however, there is considerable latitude in the use of the word—aphasia. It is a coined word which by derivation means loss of speech and some dictionaries still confine it to this narrow meaning. In the earlier medical literature it was expanded to cover not only loss of ability to speak but loss of the ability to understand the spoken word, although often these two conditions were differentiated by the use of the qualifying adjectives, motor and sensory, respectively. Because, presumably, of the very close interlinking of the various fractions of the language faculty, a still wider expansion of its meaning has since occurred so that many medical writers of today use it as a broad general term to cover all losses in the use of language including reading and writing as well as speaking and understanding speech. This is quite generally the use which is implied when the word is found in the plural as "the aphasias," while its use in the singular form, generally though not consistently, indicates a restriction of its meaning to the field of spoken language.

There are certain of the syndromes which occur in the broad general group of the aphasias which interest us specifically here because of the close similarity in the symptoms which they show to those exhibited by certain children who suffer from delays or disabilities in acquisition of language. In presenting these syndromes it must be borne in mind that they can be described here only in skeleton form and, moreover, that due to the overlapping of lesions and the interdependence of functions, *pure* cases of these conditions are exceedingly rare if indeed they occur at all in the adult, so that the descriptions given here must be considered somewhat of an abstraction. Again, while we no longer adhere to the strict "pigeonholing" of a function in a given brain area which characterized the earlier studies of the aphasias, but today think in terms of a much wider interplay of various parts of the brain, nevertheless we do recognize that given areas of the cortex may play a predominant part in language understanding and expression and that damage to such an area in the dominant hemisphere will disturb the physiological process underlying a particulate fraction of the language process to a much greater extent than it does that of the associated fractions. In this sense, localization of areas critical for different parts of the language function is therefore not only possible but serviceable and from this viewpoint such areas will be nominated with each syndrome discussed.

1. Alexia (Word Blindness)

The first of these syndromes to be reviewed is that of alexia or acquired word blindness. In this condition an individual who has previously been able to read and to write may suddenly lose both of these skills due to damage to the brain, providing that damage occurs in exactly the right locus and in the controlling or dominant hemisphere. The term "word blindness" is to some degree misleading since the individual who has suffered such a loss can still see the word but the grasp at sight of the meaning of the word is gone. Because of the location of the critical area whose destruction results in word blindness or alexia, there is very commonly a hemianopsia or loss of one half of the peripheral or scanning vision. This is not always true, however, and even in those cases in which it exists, central or macular vision which is predominately used for reading is intact and all other functions of vision except the recognition of words at sight are unaffected. Thus there is no loss in the ability to recognize the meaning and implications of objects, pictures, diagrams, etc., other than words. In brief, word blindness consists in a very highly selective loss of the capacity to recognize at a glance constellations of printed or written letters which before the injury carried with them a specific meaning. Most cases of word blindness can read the individual letters of the word and an occasional patient, by reading each letter aloud and recalling what that sequence of letters spells, may be able to identify some words, but looking at the word as a whole brings no prompt understanding of its meaning.

It is not uncommon to find that the patient suffering from word blindness cannot write but yet has not lost his skill in handwriting. The apparent paradox of this statement disappears when we learn that the patient cannot produce anything of his own composition in writing, but has in no way lost his mastery of the writing act since he can copy with ease from the production of another. Such a copy can be made from either script or print and will be produced without hesitation or tremulousness and will conform in all its individual characteristics to the writing of the patient before the brain injury occurred. The outline of alexia as here given is that of a severe case, but many partial or less severe cases are encountered, and even in the severe cases some measure of spontaneous recovery or improvement under appropriate methods of retraining may occur so that a wide range of variation in the degree of the degradation of the reading function may be observed, and some of these are instructive for our purpose. One such variant is that of the individual who can recognize many words at sight and yet has a striking defect in perception of minor differences in form, so that prefixes and suffixes tend to be disregarded or misread. Such patients also have a tendency to omit entirely all the shorter words so that the sentences as read are devoid of conjunctions, articles, prepositions, etc. Other cases may be able to read not only all the letters in a word but can recognize at sight, as an isolated unit, practically every word of moderately difficult material but have great difficulty in grasping the meaning of the sequence of words which constitute the sentence or short paragraph, particularly if the sentences be long or their structure at all unusual.

Problems in Children

Spelling as a rule is well-nigh impossible for the patient suffering from word blindness. Oral spelling is apt to be somewhat better retained than written, but large individual variations apparently enter here which may be due to the method by which a given patient was taught spelling originally. In one of the writer's cases the patient had learned to spell in boyhood almost exclusively by the oral method with much competitive recitation of the nature of "spelling bees" in school, and he had retained a considerable measure of this skill orally although his written efforts were crowded with errors in spelling and many of these were of such degree as to warrant the use of the term neographisms to describe the result.

While, as explained above, no area of the brain can be designated as the "center for reading" because of the complexity of the symptoms in every case of alexia, we can nevertheless nominate an area in the dominant hemisphere whose integrity is essential to maintaining a normal reading skill, and this critical area for this fraction of the language function is the angular gyrus and its immediate environs. (Fig. 3-1)

2. *Auditory Aphasia (Word Deafness)*

A second syndrome of the aphasias which is of particular interest to us is that of auditory aphasia or acquired word deafness. This, again, is a condition resulting from damage to the brain, but only if it affects the dominant hemisphere and is characterized by a loss of the ability to understand the spoken word in persons who have previously been competent in this regard. Acquired word deafness is a part of the some-

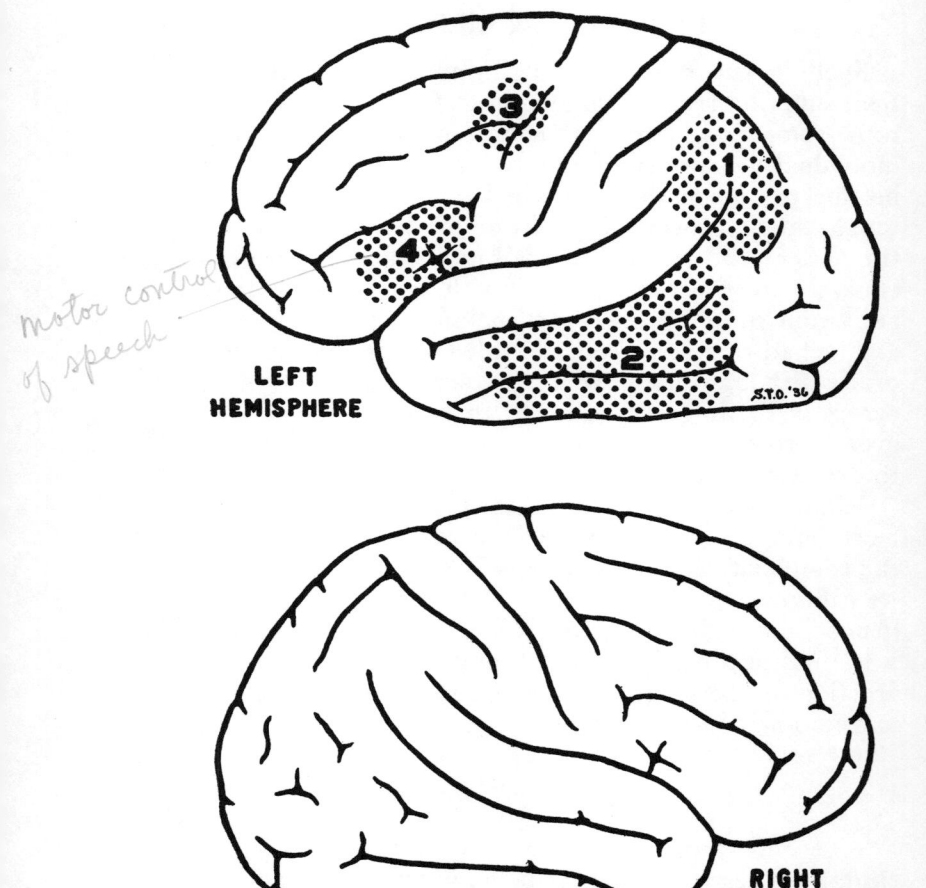

FIGURE 3. *A map of the outer surfaces of the left and right hemispheres of a human brain showing the "critical" language areas. This diagram shows the conditions as they exist in a right-handed individual, with the critical areas for language in the left hemisphere only. The four areas are defined in the text.*

Problems in Children

what broader syndrome of sensory aphasia and its existence as a pure or isolated condition is to be questioned. However, many sensory aphasics show a more or less complete loss of the ability to understand the speech of others although their hearing is intact. In such cases it is frequently possible to demonstrate by the audiometer that there is no loss either in acuity or range in the auditory function, and moreover a patient with complete loss of the understanding of words may still be able to interpret properly all other sounds of the environment such as the dinner bell, telephone ring, fire alarm, etc., and often apparently derives considerable pleasure from music. In the past there has been very little systematized testing of this stage of the auditory process and the opinion of most observers of aphasia cases as to the integrity of the function of understanding sounds rests on observations of the patient's reaction to casual noises of the environment. To meet the parallel need existing in the examination of the hearing function in children we devised, as a part of the Language Research Project of the New York Neurological Institute, a set of four phonograph records containing thirty-two commonly encountered sounds so that a more methodical examination of the competence of this function may be made. As a natural corollary of the loss of recognition of spoken words we consistently find in the sensory aphasic a striking distortion in the ability to reproduce speech properly and a very wide range of errors in the words spoken, with frequent misuse of words or mutilations which may even result in a completely unintelligible gibberish—jargon aphasia. Many of these patients can echo words after the examiner although without understanding them, thus conforming with the ability of the cases of acquired word blindness to copy in writing what they cannot read. The motor speech apparatus is intact in the patient with acquired word deafness and such cases are apt to be garrulous in spite of the fact that their efforts to express themselves rarely carry the desired meaning to their hearers. As these patients are completely cut off from the understanding of both their own speech and that of others and are almost equally handicapped in their expression of their thoughts and desires, it is almost impossible to determine in how far the intelligence suffers, but most observers consider that there gradually ensues a true intellectual degradation or dementia although many skills and acquired adaptive reactions may be preserved. In acquired word deafness, as in its counterpart in the visual function which we have already discussed, we find many cases in which the symptoms are less severe than those described above and some of the more severe cases undergo some improvement, so that again here, as in alexia, we find an almost endless variation in the degree of the patient's handicap. In the word-deaf cases, in contrast to the situation found in true organic deafness, raising the voice is of no value. Slow speech delivery and clear enunciation are, however, of major aid to the patient, as is the presentation of ideas, questions and commands in simple grammatical form and in short sentences. Such patients are occasionally able to understand individual words quite well but will fail to follow the meaning when such words are combined into phrases or sentences, or they may grasp short simple sentences correctly but lose the thread when the sentences are longer or more complex grammatically. They can at times carry out each of a number of simple commands if given separately but will become confused if they are given a series of such things to do. With many aphasic patients especial trouble is encountered in using certain word categories as, for example, the pronouns or the prepositions, or they may have difficulty with the comparatives. With others the nouns may make the most trouble—nominal aphasia. Kleist has designated as paragrammatism the type of errors seen in one form of sensory aphasia which is characterized by confusion in the use and order of words and grammatical forms, and Head has called attention to the frequent slurring or complete elision of the smaller words such as articles or conjunctions.

The area of the brain which is accepted by practically all investigators as the critical area for the understanding of words and sentences occupies the second and third temporal gyri. (Fig. 3-2)

The two foregoing groups of the aphasias affect largely, as has been emphasized in their description, the receptive apparatus for words in the field of vision and audition respectively, and result primarily in a loss of the ability to recognize the printed or the spoken word, with secondary or resultant distortions of expression in writing or in speech. These are hence called sensory language disorders, but other losses may occur which lie predominantly or exclusively in executive or expressive control of graphic or verbal language, and these are spoken of as motor disorders of the language function. As with the sensory types, a lesion of the brain involving a single hemisphere is sufficient to cause the motor language losses, but only if that lesion involve the dominant hemisphere.

3. Motor Agraphia

Many authorities question the existence of pure motor agraphia, or loss of the ability to write restricted to the expressive or motor component of this function. Unquestionably part of this doubt rests on an anatomical basis since the critical area for writing is located within a fraction of an inch of the centers which control voluntary movement of the lower arm and hand and only a short distance from the motor speech areas, and few lesions are so circumscribed and so located as to involve the critical area for writing without causing some paralysis of the writing hand or some disturbance of speech or both. However we do see cases in which there is little or no disturbance of speech and in which the actual paralysis of the master hand is too little to account for the extensive loss of writing skill, and yet in which there is no loss in the sensory side of graphic language—that is, no disturbance in the ability to recognize words at sight and to read understandingly, and which can therefore be said to be predominantly cases of motor agraphia although complicated to some degree by a greater or less amount of actual paralysis. Because of the presence of some measure of loss of muscular strength in the hand it is difficult to determine in how far skilled movements of the master hand other than writing are disordered in these cases, but coarser movements of all sorts can be carried out without difficulty and there is some evidence to show that inability to write may be a very highly selective loss not accompanied by the loss of other skills of the hand. The patient with motor agraphia, in contrast to that form of writing disorder which accompanies acquired word blindness, cannot copy, and such letters as he produces in attempts at writing are tremulous and malformed. Oral spelling is not disturbed in cases of this type and one of the writer's patients was able to arrange the letters of the game "anagrams" with sufficient accuracy to indicate that there was no disturbance of his ability in graphic spelling.

The critical area in motor agraphia is described as occupying the posterior portions of the second frontal gyrus and probably parts of the adjacent cortex on the precentral gyrus. (Fig. 3-3)

4. *Motor Aphasia*

A second disorder of the motor or expressive mechanism of the language faculty is motor aphasia. This is more or less complete speechlessness but without disorder of the peripheral speech mechanism. Again, because of the close juxtaposition of the critical area for this function and those for writing and for control of voluntary motion of the face, arm and hand, cases of disorder in the motor control of speech are commonly complicated by loss of writing and more or less paralysis of the face and hand. When the paralysis involves the muscles used in the various speech acts, an additional element of difficulty in speaking is injected. Paralysis, however, either of the master hand or of the face is not always present in motor aphasia, and frequently it is fugacious and clears up entirely soon after the injury, leaving the motor aphasia more or less in isolation. In contrast to the speech disorder which accompanies a sensory aphasia there is no loss of understanding of the spoken word and while the patient in his efforts to speak often makes use of the wrong word he is usually instantly cognizant of his error and attempts a correction. Except in complicated cases due to extensive lesions there is no loss in reading skill. Writing is frequently lost, but when this is so the disorder is of the motor type and probably due to an involvement of adjacent cortical fields. The patient suffering from motor aphasia as a rule is rather quiet and shows none of the flow of unintelligible jargon which is so apt to mark the sensory aphasic. Echo speech is usually impossible but even in severe cases with almost complete loss of speech for purposeful expression there may be considerable retention of expletives, profanity and words which have come to be associated with the expression of emotion. As a rule, however, these words are produced only under the stimulus of emotional strain. Not infrequently the motor aphasic will retain a few speech sounds or a word or phrase which is produced at almost every attempt at expressive speech. Again, as in the other forms of language disorder, all degrees of the difficulty are to be observed in a series of cases of varying severity or as spontaneous or stimulated improvement occurs. In extreme cases even the speech sounds symbolized by individual letters are lost, but more commonly these sounds can be given as an echo to the examiner or can be called when the printed letter is exhibited, but the formation of words by the blending of such sounds is arduous or impossible. In still milder

Problems in Children

degrees of the disorder many words can be spoken but the construction of sentences is difficult or impossible. This is the condition which Kleist has called "sentence muteness" and the patient's product is apt to lack many connecting words, giving rise to what the French have called "telegram style" in speech and what the Germans describe as agrammatism.

There is general agreement among students of aphasia that the critical cortex for the motor control of speech is that of Broca's area which is the posterior end of the third frontal convolution. (Fig. 3-4)

5. Apraxia

One further syndrome which will be discussed very briefly here is that of apraxia, which is the loss of a previously acquired ability to carry out intricate skilled acts. As already mentioned, a high degree of manual dexterity is one of man's marks of superiority and, as is the case with the language function, it is so organized in the brain that a unilateral lesion of the dominant hemisphere may lead to a marked degradation in skill. In one of the writer's patients there was a complete loss of the previously acquired ability in the use of the typewriter by the sense of position of the various keys. The patient could still compose the material of a letter, could spell correctly and could hunt out by eye each individual letter on the keyboard and thus make use of the instrument, but her previously acquired and highly cultivated skill in finding the keys with all fingers and without search was gone.

The parietal lobe and particularly those parts of it lying just in front of the angular gyrus region are widely accepted as the critical area for apraxic disturbances. This area is not differentially marked in the illustration.

LATERALITY—(HANDEDNESS, EYEDNESS, ETC.)

In the adult the foregoing syndromes occur almost without exception only when the injury has occurred in that half of the brain which is opposite to the master hand. Indeed, except when a stroke has occurred or other symptoms point to the locus of the lesion, we have no guide whatsoever as to which is the dominant hemisphere except the "laterality" of the individual, that is, his handedness, eyedness and footedness.

The infant at birth starts with no unilateral superiority in control of either hand or language as far as we can determine. This is supported by the entire indifference with which a very young infant uses either hand and by Pierre Marie's observation that there is no greater incidence of speech disorder in children who have suffered a birth paralysis involving the right hand than when it involves the left. Marie inferred from this that neither the right nor the left hemisphere is exclusively predestined for control of speech at birth and that if one be damaged the other can take over complete control. Most children do, however, without much question, carry an hereditary tendency to develop the predominant use of either the right or the left hemisphere. This is borne out by genetic studies of the occurrence of handedness in families and by the persistent appearance of left-handed individuals in all races in spite of many generations of directive training and strong social pressures toward the right hand, and by the relative proportion of left- and right-handedness in the general population which conforms quite closely to that which would be expected if the tendency toward right-handedness serves as a dominant heritable factor in the Mendelian sense.

Handedness, however, is so freely open to the influence of training that the resultant patterns which one finds are a combination of the hereditary bent and the effects of training. Both of these factors will vary in degree. We know today from experimental genetics that it is only when crossings of homozygous or pure stocks take place that the typical Mendelian segregation of opposite characters occurs. When crossings are not between pure stocks but rather include a long series of matings which are promiscuous so far as a given set of opposing characters is concerned, varying degrees of intermingling of these characters will occur which are technically known as "intergrades." Obviously the question of handedness has not entered into human matings in the past and we might therefore anticipate intermixtures between right- and left-sidedness which we call "motor intergrades."

Not only will the hereditary tendency toward use of the right or left hand vary with the degree of this process of intergrading, but the training which each such individual receives is also a highly variable factor. For the most part this tends to lead the individual toward the right hand, first, because the great majority of people are right-handed and naturally assume that their children are also going to be, and second, because there exists no inconsiderable amount of prejudice against left-handedness, which in many instances is so strong as to amount to the belief that the left-hander is abnormal. This prejudice is reflected in the derived meanings of the Latin word "sinister" and the French "gauche." There is certainly no justification for this belief and there is reason to believe that a high degree of specialization in either hemisphere makes for superiority and that the good left-hander is therefore not only not abnormal but is apt to be better equipped than is the indifferent right-hander. The rigor of training to which a left-handed child is exposed is also a great variable extending all the way from simple measures such as transferring the spoon from the left to the right hand while the child is learning to eat to more drastic procedures such as tying up the left hand so that the right must be used. It is rare indeed that training is exerted to produce a left-handed individual, but three cases have come to the writer's attention where this was true. One was an instance in which the mother herself became confused while facing the child across the table as to which was the child's right hand, and persistently insisted on the use of the spoon and other implements in the child's left hand. The other two were both boys who were trained from early childhood toward left-handedness by their fathers with the intent of developing them into baseball pitchers. Neither boy succeeded in acquiring a good left-handed pitching skill.

We will exclude from this discussion those cases in which disease or accident to the brain in childhood has brought about an early shift of the handedness pattern, since they form an exceptional group by reason of the fact that the integrity of the brain structure has been altered and the shift is usually to be looked upon as the result of a preferential use of the least damaged

Problems in Children

side of the brain. Accident to the hand or arm, however, or infantile paralysis, which does not involve the brain, not infrequently enforces a change in handedness which is quite comparable in its results to that brought about by enforced training, since there is here no change in the integrity of the brain mechanisms, and we have seen complications associated with shift of handedness so caused quite comparable to those which may follow efforts to change the natural handedness of a child by disciplinary and training methods.

STUDIES IN LATERALITY

While our whole knowledge of unilateral cerebral dominance rests on the study of the aphasias and subsequent investigation of the brain, yet, as suggested above, we are limited in our clinical studies of children to observations of the laterality of the child, and these have been found to be much less easy than might have been anticipated. We are accustomed to think in terms of clear cut preferences for the right or the left hand and it would seem, therefore, that a determination of the preferred hand would be a relatively easy matter. Our findings, however, do not conform to this and it has become necessary to use a battery of tests, and even when these have been applied the interpretation of the examiner based upon his experience with a considerable number of children is often necessary before a conclusion can be reached.

There are three factors entering into the question of laterality—eyedness, footedness and handedness. Eyedness, or the selection of one or the other eye chosen whenever the individual is compelled to use only one, as in looking through a knothole in a fence, for example, is not so widely recognized as handedness but it is probably of equal importance. It is not so susceptible to training but the writer has so far encountered at least one case in which there was a clear cut story of a purposeful shift in eyedness. This was an instance in which a boy found himself in difficulty in using the rifle because of his right-handedness and left-eyedness. Since eyedness is not so readily affected by training some have thought this to be a better guide to the inherent or native sidedness than is the master hand. Parson, particularly, championed this viewpoint and went so far as to hold that all left-eyed and right-handed individuals were native left-handers who had been shifted by training, and further held that the sighting eye determined the master hand. Unfortunately for this thesis it does not explain the group with the obverse pattern—those who are left-handed and right-eyed, nor does it explain the large number of individuals who do not have a strong predilection for either eye in sighting. Extensive studies in eyedness in the past few years have brought us to the belief that no one test is to be trusted, and have also demonstrated that there exists a complete and graduated series from the strongly right-eyed to the strongly left-eyed individual, with all stages and degrees of amphiocularity represented in between. We have used quite a wide variety of tests of eyedness—toy microscope, toy telescope, peep-hole toys, hole-in-card test, kaleidoscope, Miles' V-scope, Parson's manoptoscope, etc., and have come to the conclusion that no one test can be said to be entirely trustworthy and that some such wide battery as that listed here must be used. One of the tests most extensively used and often exclusively depended upon in psychological laboratories, that is, Parson's manoptoscope, has proven in our hands the least trustworthy and the most apt to be at variance with the other tests of the battery. Those tests of the series in which one hand is used to raise the test object, i.e., the telescope, kaleidoscope, peep-toys, etc., bring in the factor of handedness which may apparently in amphiocular cases lead to a choice of the corresponding eye. As a balance against this, the hole-in-card test has been used with the card held first by the examiner for several trials and with the hole as nearly in front of the bridge of the nose as possible. After this, the card is held by the patient first in his right hand, then in his left and finally in both hands. Not infrequently this will reveal the influence of the hand used, as when the card is brought to the right eye with the right hand and to the left eye with the left and with neither eye promptly chosen when both hands are used.

Gould believed that the eye with the better vision determines a superiority of the corresponding hand and claimed that the right eye has the better acuity in 94% of all infants and that this determines the high proportion of right- as compared with left-handedness. Our own findings do not permit of comment on Gould's statement concerning infants but we have encountered a number of cases of children in whom definitely poorer vision was demonstrable not only on the side corresponding to the handedness but in the eye used for sighting, that is, the master eye, as well and, moreover, as Wile has pointed out, Ballard's statement, that the same proportion of right- and left-handedness occurs among the congenitally blind as among the seeing, is a trenchant objection to both Gould's and Parson's belief. Some anatomists have called attention to the frequency with which the occipital pole—the visual sphere—of the brain is apparently somewhat larger on the left than on the right, and this has been held to be in support of the view that visual dominance precedes and may determine handedness. In the writer's experience this has not proven a dependable guide and one factor which may be misleading here is the very frequent distortion from a true ellipsoidal outline which is to be found in human skulls and brains. In many instances where one occipital pole seems to be better developed, a compensatory bulge will be found in the contralateral frontal pole suggesting strongly that the whole brain is somewhat askew and that the better development of the occipital region on one side may be more apparent than real. This distortion sometimes favors one side and sometimes the other but again as far as the writer's observations go, it does not correlate with the handedness of the individual.

It is interesting to note that in spite of the extended discussion which has been given to the problem of the master eye, almost all observers have been thinking in terms of visual acuity and almost no attention has been given to the fact that using the eye for sighting is primarily a function of motor control rather than of vision. To sight, we attempt to bring the center of the macula, the pupil and the object of regard into line, and quite obviously this is an act dependent much more directly on the skillful use of the extraocular muscles than it is on the clarity with which the object itself be seen, unless indeed there be very marked differences in the visual competence on the two sides. This view of ocular dominance conforms to our findings that unless the difference in refractive errors be great they play little apparent part in the choice of a master eye and that the eye preferred for sighting may actually have the greater error. Consideration of the dominant eye as dependent on the more ready use of the ocular muscles on one side brings this subject into immediate and close relation with the greater muscular skill developed by the master hand and limits interpretations based on vague concepts of visual superiority.

Footedness is not so important as eyedness and handedness, although fixed patterns of selective choice are not infrequently found in hopping, kicking a football, starting up a flight of steps, mounting a bicycle, using the coaster brake, etc., and when such selective choices occur they are generally, although not consistently, on the same side as the master hand.

In studies of the handedness of an individual, both history and tests are of importance. We have made it a practice to take a history of the developmental period from the parents or others who have been associated with the child at this stage, and also to question the patient himself with regard to his current practices, asking him to demonstrate whenever possible his choice of hand in everyday activities such as the use of a comb, toothbrush, eating utensils, baseball bat, tennis racquet, saw, hammer and other tools and implements. Both types of histories may be instructive although they are occasionally misleading or contrary. From the parent, inquiry is made concerning three points in particular: first, whether there was any delay in establishing a choice of a preferred hand beyond the period when the average child makes such a selection; second, whether any efforts, rigorous or mild, were made to encourage or enforce the use of either hand, and third, whether the patient showed any undue clumsiness in acquiring such skills as buttoning clothes, tying shoelaces, using eating utensils, etc. Occasionally a parent has become somewhat sensitive concerning earlier efforts to direct the child's handedness and is not quite frank concerning the measures adopted, but much more commonly the history is misleading because of poor observation. In one such case a child, who proved both by observation and by test to be electively left-handed in everything except three activities in which he had been definitely trained, was reported by his mother to be entirely right-handed. His mother came of a family with considerable left-handedness and had no prejudice against it and I believe was entirely sincere in this statement. And, moreover, his nurse had also entirely overlooked the fact that he preferred his left hand. Because of this factor it is sometimes advisable to plan a period of observation of the child in his home for a week or more during which the parents are instructed to watch him with care and to note particularly his preferences in those acts in which he has not received instruction.

Occasionally the child's training has been left so entirely in the hands of a nurse or maid who has later left the family's employ that it is impossible to get a history of the early development and the parents are quite unaware as to whether an effort has been made to change his spontaneous handedness tendency. The fact that left-handedness has often been associated in the minds of the uneducated with misfortune, as in the Irish use of the word *kithogue* is to be remembered

Problems in Children

here and many nurses will, on their own responsibility, attempt to ward off such evil from their charges. In the case of older children or in large families, the parents' memory is usually increasingly unreliable and the patient's own history should then be taken to determine his actual preferences in all sorts of activities in which one hand alone is used. Here we find the effects of training are very much to the fore and frequently the child will remember definite efforts on the part of some adult to establish one or the other pattern for him in certain selected activities. Thus one boy, who is a confirmed sinistral in all activities except golf, tells of the difficulty he had in learning this game because no left-handed clubs were available and he also adds, quite pertinently, "It is my poorest sport." Occasionally mere example will suffice to fix the right- or left-hand pattern. This was strikingly brought home to the writer by the story of a friend in the West who during his college days made quite a name for himself as a pole vaulter. He was entirely right-sided—hand, foot and eye—except for his pole vaulting in which he used the left-hand position. To account for this he described his first contact with this sport. A group of athletes gave an exhibition in his home town during his senior year in high school and among them was a pole vaulter who happened to be left-handed. The observing boy was instantly enamored of this sport and throughout the summer, in imagination only, was running down the field carrying the vaulting pole in the left-hand position. When in the following fall he entered college, the track coach, finding him right-handed in other things, made vigorous efforts to teach him the right-hand position in vaulting, but to no avail. He had so fixed the motor pattern during his summer of contemplation that the substitution of the other was impossible and the coach ultimately gave up his efforts and let him go forward as a left-handed vaulter. This history is recited primarily to show the relatively small amount of influence which is required to cause a change in pattern in some individuals and hence the insecurity of an opinion based on other than extended tests, history and observation.

Occasionally a child is encountered who is so obviously eager to prove to the examiner that he is entirely right-handed that the account which he gives of his own preferences and even his showing on the tests must be discounted to some extent. Such an attitude does, however, suggest strongly that someone in his environment has influenced him in favor of the right-sided pattern. Again, children who are neither predominantly right- nor left-handed may have an unusual amount of difficulty in learning which is right and which is left, and their verbal account of their handedness preferences may be at striking variance with a simultaneous demonstration of their habitual choices. Many are conscious of this confusion and will give a history of difficulty in following directions involving turns to the right and to the left.

As a compliment to the history of past development and recognized preferences, tests of current skills are of importance to establish the actual status of the moment. Quite a wide variety of tests may be employed, even for comparatively young children. Throwing movements, both those of the overarm throw and the underarm toss, are of value in showing the relative facility of use of the muscles of the shoulders and upper arms of the two sides. Tests such as putting pegs in holes, counting with the finger push comptometer, and others of this general nature should also be included to determine the relative skills of the two hands in such movements and also so that a comparison may be made between the skills of the shoulder and arm movements and those of the hand and fingers. At the same time observations should be made as to the relative degree of ease and grace in carrying out these activities. In order to minimize the effect of training we have found it wise to include in the battery of motor tests an element of novelty free from the effects of training or practice as far as this is possible, and we have devised and adapted apparatus for this purpose, but if the choice of tests in common activities be broad enough they seem to meet the need as well as more elaborate apparatus.

Many statements are to be found in the literature concerning the superior strength in the master hand, and this has been tested by the use of a pair of dynamometers used first simultaneously in the two hands and then one at a time in each hand. We have found no consistent relation between strength of arm and the master hand except when the latter has been well established and has long done the major part of the manual work, and we consider this factor too unstable to be of value.

For a time it was hoped that an electrical study of the action currents of the forearm would prove a dependable guide to the inherent or native handedness pattern of a given individual. This was based on the work of Golla in London who, by using two galvanometers, found in a left-handed individual that there was a tendency of the action currents of the left arm to precede in time those of the right when both hands were closed simultaneously. Travis and the writer carried out some further observations along this line on a small series of stutterers and normal speakers some years ago in the Iowa Psychopathic Hospital with what looked at the time like very promising results. A much larger series has now been studied including pure right- and left-handed individuals and some who were left-handed in all spontaneous activities but used the right for certain trained skills, notably writing, and including individuals with and without various types of language disorders. In this study much better instruments were provided in the laboratories of the Language Research Unit of the New York Neurological Institute, and not only was the series of cases investigated much larger and more carefully selected but the number of readings in each case was considerably greater. The results were disappointing in that it was found that while Golla's formula of a slight precedence in time of arrival of the action currents on the master side was often correct, yet there were so many exceptions that the use of this test to determine the inherent pattern in any given individual could not be depended upon and the method has had to be discarded as a diagnostic procedure. It is to be noted, however, that this method which is dependent on readings of the action currents in the forearm is subject to several uncontrollable sources of possible error, and that direct registration of the electrical activity in various brain areas such as is made possible by the new electroencephalograph offers promise of excluding these errors and may give us trustworthy and valuable results in this and certain kindred problems in the language disorders.

MOTOR INTERGRADING

A large number of children have now been studied with extensive histories and by batteries of tests for both eye and hand preferences. Most of them came from the selected group which was referred to our laboratories because of some form of developmental defect in language. This series shows quite a number who were entirely right-sided and some who were entirely left-sided, but in addition it includes a great many whose motor patterns showed a striking mixture of right- and left-sidedness. Some, for example, were right-handed and left-eyed; some left-handed and right-eyed; some indifferent in their handedness and amphiocular. In some, moreover, the large movements of the shoulders such as are used for throwing were much more skillful and graceful on the left side, while the finer movements of the hands such as are used in writing were better on the right. This is a situation which one is apt to encounter in a left-handed child who has followed his own bent in throwing but has been taught to use his right hand for writing and drawing. In still other children there was no frank intermixture of right and left patterns but much less than the amount of difference between the skills of the two sides usually found in the strongly right- or strongly left-handed individual.

Another factor which we found complicating the study of handedness preferences was that in some children in this group with mixed motor patterns, especially the younger ones, there was a striking lack of stability in their choices. The same test repeated on different days not infrequently gave opposite results, and in certain cases observation of the child in his home showed a decided preference for the left hand on some days and an equally selective choice of the right on others. Again, in several children, we have observed what appears to have been a spontaneous shift from left- to right-handedness occurring without any demonstrable external influence. This has appeared at various ages but most frequently between the ages of two and three and the ages of six and eight, which constitute the two critical periods in language development which will be discussed later in this volume.

While the majority of our cases are those of children who have come to us because of delay or disorder in the development of some phase of the language faculty, we have also carried out the same tests of handedness and eyedness on a limited number of adults who gave no history of language difficulties, and we have found instances of crossed and mixed patterns among them also, so that we feel that the occurrence of motor intergrading is by no means to be considered a fixed measure of the ability to acquire either manual or linguistic skills. It is, we believe, to be looked upon as evidence of the absence of a sufficiently strong hereditary tendency to establish a clear cut selective preference for one side in *all* motor acts but since such intergrading will include all degrees of intermixture there will be many individuals who exhibit some evidence of mixed sidedness and yet who have met with no difficulty in acquiring either complex motor acts or spoken or written language.

One of the outstanding characteristics of the individual who is endowed with a very strong tendency toward the use of either the left or the right hand is his persistence in adhering to his natural preference in spite of the environmental pressures brought to bear. Examples of this are to be seen in many left-handed people who have been forced to learn to use the right hand for writing in school but who, as soon as this pressure has been relaxed, have reverted to writing with the left hand because of greater ease and speed. When we consider this, the occurrence of a group of children who exhibit little bent toward either the right- or left-hand pattern in spite of the usual exposure to training and of another group who start with a slight preference for the left but even with the most moderate pressure are led to shift to the right, is, we believe, strong evidence that this group of mixed, crossed, and undecided patterns indicates the presence of an inherent variable here, and our findings in this selected group of children seem to be explicable only on the existence of a graded series of sidedness preference extending all the way from very strongly right-sided individuals to very strongly left-sided ones and with all degrees of intermingling in between. This is what might be anticipated as the result of intergrading between two genetic factors leading respectively to left- and right-sidedness.

Granting a striking variation in the strength of the hereditary tendency, it is obvious that the results of various training methods on different children will likewise be a variable, and this we believe is the unquestionable answer to the very wide difference of opinion which exists as to the influence of an enforced change in the child's natural handedness inclinations. A long and bitter battle has raged about this question and both extremes of opinion still find vigorous protagonists. There are those who feel that no harm can ensue from making every child conform to a right-handed pattern, and indeed in many schools today no child is permitted to write with his left hand. At the other extreme are those who feel with equal conviction that every effort at shifting a child from his natural patterns will result in some one or another sort of difficulty.

The great degree of individual variation which has become increasingly apparent as our studies of laterality have progressed makes it clear that no dogmatic general answer can be given to the question as to whether a left-handed child should ever be trained on the right side. The question can be answered only for a given individual after tests and observations of the child himself, and even then it is sometimes necessary to experiment with a period of training and, in one or two instances, such an experimental period demonstrated that our first opinion based on history and tests was not leading to the expected results in training and it was necessary to change the program completely. One other factor which must be considered here is the age of the child. As will be elaborated in a subsequent chapter, there are certain periods in a child's development—notably between two to three, and six to eight years of age—which are critical in the development of the language function, and interference with inherent handedness patterns at these times seems much more prone to give rise to difficulties than at others. There

Problems in Children

is abundant evidence, for example, that shift of handedness enforced by injury in the right arm of a right-handed adult will have no demonstrable effect on his speech, whereas a comparable situation arising during one of the two critical periods just mentioned is very apt indeed to be followed by a speech disorder.

In the group of children who, however, are clearly not developing a selective skill in either hand or in whom the balance is comparatively close, it seems highly advisable to increase definitely both the skill and the habit of use of the hand on the side which has the greater capacity, if this can be determined. When the balance is fairly equal, preference is given to the training of the right hand in most cases. Concerning those children, however, who show an early and distinct preference of their own for the use of either hand, we feel that the only logical plan is to permit them to follow this physiological bent without outside interference, which at best is probably guided largely by prejudice. One occasionally finds parents or teachers who are attempting to train a child towards complete ambidexterity, overlooking the fact that with man's development in manual skill, which we mentioned at the outset of this volume as one of his two great advances over the lower animals, we find an increasing tendency towards the preferential use of one hand or the other. Although we have seen many children who exhibit a high degree of ambivalence between the left and right hands, they have commonly shown less than the usual skill for their age in the more intricate movements of either, and we have encountered none in whom true ambidexterity could be said to exist, that is, where all skills on the two sides were not only equal but also highly developed. There seems to be a fair uniformity of opinion in the literature that the so-called ambidextrous person is usually a native sinistral who has acquired through training a considerable measure of skill in certain right-sided activities, and our experience would tend to confirm this. In many of these cases, it is true, training on the two sides has not resulted in any demonstrable harm to the individual but the much higher degree of the motor skill generally exhibited by "pure" right- and "pure" left-handers leads to the conjecture that even the very skillful ambidextrous individual might have been still more facile had he been trained electively in accordance with his natural physiological bent.

The very close parallelism which exists between the symptoms to be seen in adults who have suffered a loss in language as a result of brain injury and those to be seen during the development of the language faculty in some children suggests very strongly that we are dealing with a disturbance of the same physiological process in both instances and, since in the adult such a loss occurs only when the lesion is in the master hemisphere, our attention is naturally directed to those factors, open to our observation and study, which tend to determine the choice and establishment of unilateral brain control. For reasons which are too technical to be reviewed in detail here, the hypothesis that these developmental disorders in acquiring the language functions are the result of faulty development of particular brain areas (agenetic cortical defects) is no longer tenable, while the existence of demonstrable mixtures between right and left motor preferences with a strong familial background implies that comparable intergrading may exist between the critical areas for the various fractions of the language faculty in the two hemispheres of the brain, thus giving rise to a series of developmental disorders in language, a description of which will form Chapter Two of this volume.

Chapter Two

CERTAIN DISORDERS IN THE DEVELOPMENT OF
LANGUAGE IN CHILDREN

THE first part of this volume reviewed very briefly some of the disorders which follow small areas of destruction of the brain in the adult after language has been acquired, and it was pointed out that these losses of language occur only when the master half of the brain is affected and that the only guide we have as to whether the right or left hemisphere of the brain is operating as the master half in the normal individual is his "sidedness" as shown by his handedness, footedness and eyedness. A summary of studies in sidedness in a large number of children and adults was offered, which indicates the existence of a wide range of variability in the establishment of the master hand and eye. Since the principle of functional superiority of one brain hemisphere is operative in the control of the language function in the normal adult as well as in determining a greater capacity for the acquisition of skilled acts on one side of the body, we may safely assume that a variability exists in the establishment of the unilateral patterns in language development in the child comparable to the demonstrable variation found in the motor patterns.

Discussions in the medical literature of the past bearing on the syndromes of defect or delay in language acquisition in childhood have for the most part stressed the inherent or hereditary factors involved, and the term congenital has come into wide use to differentiate these disorders as met in the growing child from the comparable conditions which result from brain injury or brain disease in the adult which are described as acquired syndromes. While the importance of heredity is clearly recognized and accepted here, nevertheless we feel that use of the term congenital tends to overstress the inherent difficulty and to underemphasize the many environmental factors, both specific—such as methods of teaching—and more general—such as emotional and social forces—and we therefore prefer the use of the term developmental to congenital since it may be said to include both the hereditary tendency and the environmental forces which are brought to play on the individual.

DESCRIPTION OF SYNDROMES

1. Developmental Alexia (The Reading Disability)

The first of the syndromes of delay or disorder in language acquisition, encountered by certain children, to be discussed here is that of developmental alexia (congenital word blindness, strephosymbolia, specific reading disability). This was first described by Morgan in England under the name of congenital word blindness but Hinshelwood, an English opthalmologist, gave us the first intensive study of the condition in a monograph published in 1917. A number of children were referred to Hinshelwood because of their lack of progress in learning to read and because it was thought that this might be caused by some disorder in vision. This did not prove to be the case, but in his critical study of these children Hinshelwood placed emphasis on two very pertinent facts: first, that there are often several such cases in one family, and second, that the symptoms which they show are very closely parallel to those which appear in adults who have lost the capacity to read because of injury to the brain. At that time studies of the adult cases had pointed out the critical relation which the angular gyrus of the dominant hemisphere bears to loss of reading skill and this brain area was considered to be the storehouse for visual memories of words. Basing his deductions on this, Hinshelwood hypothecated a congenital defect of development (agenesis) of this particular area of the brain in such children. There has been no evidence forthcoming to support this defect hypothesis since Hinshelwood's time, and there is much to be said against it. In the first place, such areas of agenesis are of comparatively rare occurrence and are not met with in a general autopsy service with anywhere near the frequency with which the cases of reading disability are to be encountered among children. Secondly, if it be true as Marie reported that there is no higher incidence of speech disorders in children born with a right hemiplegia than in those with a left, and if Marie's assumption from this, that when one hemisphere is damaged before speech is learned the other can take its place, is correct, it would then require a lack of development in the angular gyri of both hemispheres to satisfy Hinshelwood's hypothesis, and such bilateral agenetic defects are exceedingly rare. Finally, as our studies of cerebral functioning have progressed, we have been led to discard the older concept of the angular gyrus region as a brain area in which more or less photographic visual memories of words are stored and have come to realize that the process of reading is a much more complex activity requiring the physiological integrity and interplay of many brain areas although the angular gyrus and its adjacent cortex in the dominant hemisphere still bear a critical relation to this function, as we have seen in our review of acquired alexia.

The term congenital word blindness as used in medical literature to describe the reading disability is misleading, first since it tends, as discussed above, to overemphasize the inherent factor and second since there is no true blindness in the ordinary use of this term nor, indeed, is there even blindness for words. This can be readily demonstrated by the fact that cases with severe reading disability can copy words correctly which they cannot read at all. In other words, the word is seen but not recognized. The writer, in 1926, in the course of an intensive study of several cases of this disorder noted a striking tendency to distorted order in the recall of letters shown in the attempts of these children to read a word or to spell it and offered the term strephosymbolia—meaning "twisted symbols"—as more descriptive of the symptomatic condition than is congenital word blindness.

In his monograph Hinshelwood attempted to separate the more extreme cases of reading disability and would restrict the term congenital word blindness to those in whom the difficulty in learning to read was "so great and so unusual that it could be regarded without any exaggeration as an abnormal or pathological condition." He did not, however, offer any usable criterion as to how such a separation of the pathological cases could be made, and our experience in studying and retraining several hundred such cases over a period of years has convinced us that the strephosymbolics cannot be so divided but rather that they form a graded series including all degrees of severity of the handicap.

Because of this wide variation in the expression of this disability no attempt will be made here to describe all the variants but the syndrome will be presented as seen in two very characteristic forms of the disorder: first, that of cases seen very early before the influence of training has too far altered the picture, and with them that of very severe cases where attempts at training have had little influence; and second, that of mild or residual cases where reading has been acquired but to so poor an advantage that failures in secondary school and college may be definitely referred to this educational shortcoming.

Obviously there are multiple causes for a delay in learning to read. Marked defects in vision may underlie such a difficulty and should be thoroughly investigated and, if present, corrected. Defects of hearing have also been encountered which have led to poor auditory discrimination of words and in some cases poor reading has seemed to have its roots in residuals of an uncorrected word deafness which is to be discussed later herein. General intellectual defect is also a frequent cause of failure in reading. Emotional disturbances, such as antagonisms toward a particular teacher or general apathy toward all school work, or lack of adequate disciplinary training at home, may all play their part in giving rise to a slow start in this

Problems in Children

academic need. When, however, all of such factors are excluded, there remains a group of very considerable size in every school who have shown no evidence of any delay or abnormality in either their physical, mental, or emotional development until they have reached school and are confronted with reading, and then they suddenly meet a task which they cannot accomplish.

When seen early—that is, during the first two years of exposure to reading, usually between the ages of six and eight—the earmark of the specific reading difficulty is an inability to learn to recognize words at sight as readily as do the facile readers. The more rapid learners in this field of education are no brighter on the average than are some of the reading disability cases, and indeed some of our very severe strephosymbolics when measured by all available tests rank high in intelligence. The writer, for example, has studied one boy who was reading almost nothing and spelling less, after three years in school, who passed intelligence tests with a quotient of 145 and gave every evidence in every other field except his reading, spelling and writing of being a "near genius." Thus intelligence does not always correlate with reading skill, and in any group of non-readers all ranges of intelligence are to be found as they would be in any casually selected group of children. A word of caution must be offered here, however, and that is that poor reading comprehension forms an integral part of the general picture presented by children with dull normal intelligence and those of the defective group, so that failure in learning to read with understanding must not be considered a specific disability unless it is distinctly out of harmony with the child's skill in other fields—notably the ability to learn by hearing and to master arithmetical concepts. A simple method of showing quantitatively the specific character of the retardation which occurs in children suffering from developmental alexia is by means of an educational profile on which are entered the child's grade, actual age, mental age and his accomplishment in standard tests of arithmetic, reading, spelling and writing. Three such charts are given in Figures 4, 5 and 6. Much more striking contrasts are available in our records in cases of older children suffering with extreme degrees of this disability, but such cases are relatively rare and the three presented here have been chosen to show the characteristic picture at three age levels in the more commonly encountered cases of moderate severity. In each profile, "Grade" refers to the placement given the child at school, "C.A." indicates chronological age, while "M.A." gives the mental age as determined by a Stanford-Binet examination. It will be noted that all three of these cases were children of superior intelligence, and it may be added that they came from educated families and good schools. The standings given in arithmetic, reading, and spelling were obtained by averaging two or more standardized tests in each of these subjects, and the grade in writing is that of writing speed as determined by the Ayres scale.

Usually the auditory development of these children has been quite normal. There is no defect in the acuity of hearing; they have learned to differentiate and interpret the various sounds of the environment; understanding of words has been good and they have learned to speak at about the usual age. Some indeed are ex-

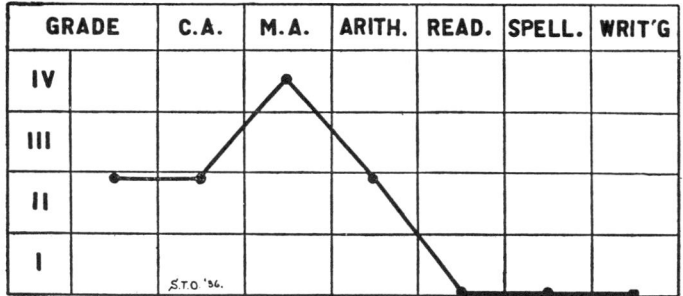

FIGURE 4. *Educational profile of an eight-year-old left-handed boy with a superior intelligence but a retardation in reading, spelling and writing, typical of strephosymbolia in younger children. C.A. indicates chronological age. M.A. indicates mental age.*

FIGURE 5. *Educational profile of a ten-year-old right-handed girl with a moderate degree of strephosymbolia. Abbreviations are the same as in Figure 4.*

ceedingly keen in the auditory field and are able to memorize pages of their readers from hearing their classmates recite, so that their own inability in reading may be hidden from the teachers for a time. As they

GRADE	C.A.	M.A.	ARITH.	READ.	SPELL.	WRIT'G
VIII						
VII						
VI						
V						
IV						
III						
II						
I						

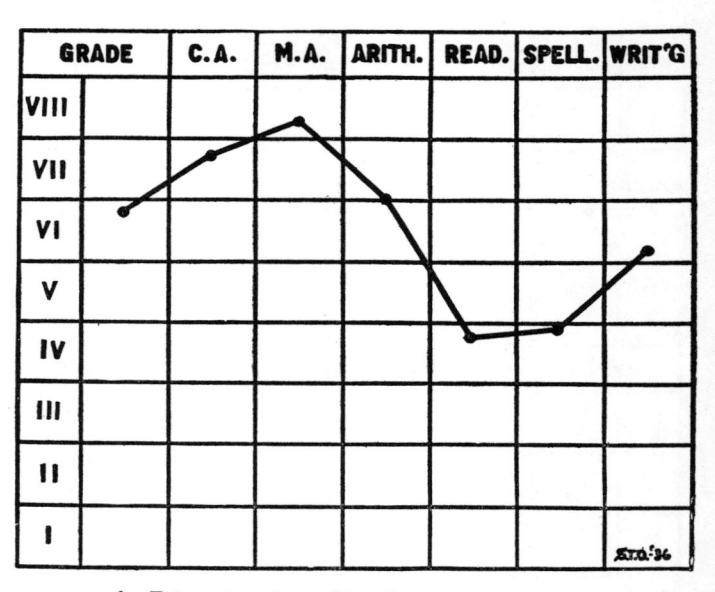

FIGURE 6. *Educational profile of a fourteen-year-old right-handed girl with a moderate degree of strephosymbolia. Abbreviations are the same as in Figure 4.*

progress, however, they outrun this skill and it soon becomes apparent that the word which they see does not bring recognition in spite of the many times which it has been shown to them. Under such circumstances, reading very often takes on largely the qualities of a game of guessing at words, or the child will offer a word with no likeness in form or suitability in context to that which he is attempting to read. Sometimes, indeed, a highly imaginative child will concoct a whole story bearing no relation to the words on the page before him beyond one or two initial or key words which he cleverly weaves into his own production. In very severe cases, the child may remain practically at this level for years unless appropriate methods of training are adopted. Such children are usually avidly interested in stories, both those told to them and those read aloud, and although this is a valuable means of developing their auditory vocabulary and providing factual data of which they would otherwise be deprived because of their lack of reading ability, a difficulty sometimes enters here in that much reading aloud is apt to develop the interests of such a youngster far beyond the point which he will be able to reach in reading for himself for several years.

Vision in the group of non-readers at large is not defective. Minor errors of refraction and muscle imbalance are encountered here as they would be in any group of children but no more frequently, and some of our extreme cases of strephosymbolia have vision which is far better than the average of those who are learning to read with ease. We have not had the opportunity to check the strephosymbolics from the standpoint of relative size of the retinal images in the two eyes (aniseikonia) but we feel that the demonstrable fact that their difficulty lies in recalling previous exposures of the word rather than in seeing it, permits the practical exclusion of this factor as of importance. Our observations on the presence of suspenopsia and on the capacity for binocular fusion and stereopsis show no consistent deviation in the children with a reading disability from the normal variation to be found in these functions in good readers.

Functions other than reading but which incorporate a visual element are usually entirely normal. For example, visuo-motor co-ordination may be excellent as is shown by superiority in various games requiring close control of movement by vision, such as baseball or tennis, and by the interest and ability which the strephosymbolic frequently shows in intricate handwork. Visual recognition of objects, of places, and of persons is quite normal, and interpretation of pictorial and diagrammatic material is frequently very good. Sense of direction is also often well developed as in the case of one boy with such a marked reading difficulty that he could not understand any of the signboards along the way, who had nevertheless memorized routes so that he was the trusted family guide for automobile trips.

That there is no true blindness for words as the older nomenclature would suggest is clearly emphasized by the fact that these children see the word and will make an attempt to read it although such an effort commonly does not bring correct recognition, and this is still further brought into relief by the fact that many of these non-readers are able to copy correctly words which they cannot read. This is particularly well demonstrated in certain instances by asking the child to copy and later to read short nonsense syllables in which the element of past exposure and hence an unknown measure of familiarity does not enter. Even the confusing *b*'s and *d*'s are copied perfectly although often presenting a hopeless confusion when read.

While the early cases of strephosymbolia and those

Problems in Children

of more extreme severity often have learned to read very little indeed, nevertheless an observation of the type of errors which they make in attempting to read is instructive. In the beginning we find a very wide range of letter confusions—b's are mixed with h's; m, n and u are confused, etc. Such confusion is present in practically all children in the very beginning but the more facile readers very quickly straighten them out and even the reading disability cases, with a little teaching, soon get most of the letters properly associated with their names, with the notable exception of those letters which are similar in form but reversed in orientation, that is, b and d, and p and q. In some of our more confused cases difficulty has been encountered in telling t from f, and a from s. This will be more readily understood if the imprint of the lower case type for these letters is examined in the mirror, as this brings out similarities which might quite escape us otherwise. Not infrequently children who have been struggling with their b's and d's and have learned to tell them apart when they are isolated may easily be led to exhibit their uncertainty by the exposure of a word containing one of these "twin letters" but which otherwise is like that of a more familiar word which contains the other. Thus children who have often seen the word "big" but are not so well acquainted with "dig" will often read both as "big." As a rule b and d, being more frequently met, are more readily straightened out, and it is not uncommon to find a child who can differentiate these two letters in all except the most treacherous associations but who still has trouble with p and q, and indeed it may be fair to raise the question as to whether this confusion may not have given rise to the admonition "to mind your *p*'s and *q*'s."

In the poor readers, reversible words also form a serious stumbling block; "was" and "saw," "on" and "no," "not" and "ton," are inextricably mixed. There is also a marked tendency to twist around a pair of letters in a word, leading to confusion between such words as "from" and "form"; "calm" and "clam," etc. Or occasionally the reversal of one syllable of a word occurs as when "tarnish" is read as "tarshin" or "ratnish," or there may be a reversed assembly of two syllables of a word, each of which has been read in the proper direction, as when "repast" is read as "ast-rep." One striking fact about this reversal tendency is its instability. The letter *b* is sometimes *b* and sometimes *d;* "was" encountered several times in the same paragraph may come back as either "was" or "saw" with no consistency. As the child grows older and progresses somewhat in his ability to solve these puzzles of direction, and especially when he begins to make use of the context to determine his choices between two possibilities, the use of three- and four-letter nonsense syllables and combinations constructed of two, three, or four such syllables will frequently uncover a tendency to reversals which has to a considerable extent disappeared from familiar words. While these errors are to be observed by listening to the child's reading, they can be graphically shown in written productions to good advantage. Figures 7 and 8 are examples. In Figure 7, the boy attempted, when writing the alphabet from memory, to dodge the confusion between the lower case forms of *b* and *d* by using capitals. When asked to write the small letters,

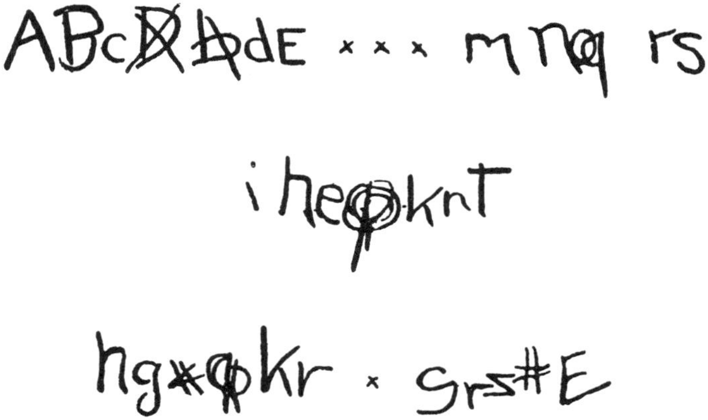

FIGURE 7. *Graphic evidence of the confusion between* b *and* d *and* p *and* q *in the writing of an eight-year-old boy with a marked reading disability.*

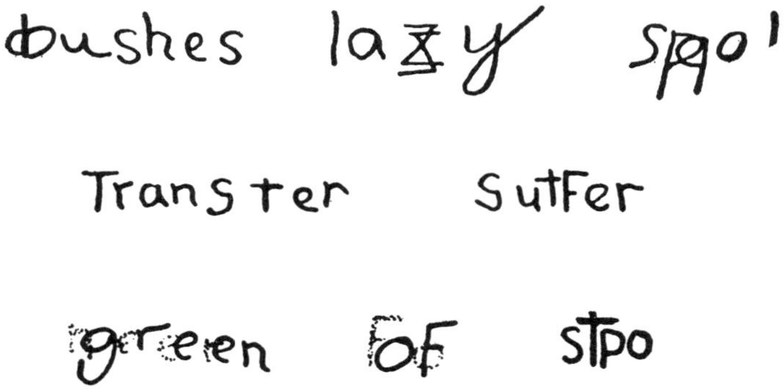

FIGURE 8. *Confusion in the orientation of letters and in direction of writing from the work of a ten-year-old strephosymbolic girl.*

he produced a *b* for a *d* but saw his error and corrected it. When he came to *p* and *q*, he fired both barrels at once and had to omit the second of this pair. In writing to dictation of the letter names the fourth symbol in the second row was produced when *p* was dictated, and this also applies to the corresponding symbol which appears in the bottom row when he was writing letters in response to dictated sounds. In Figure 8, the difficulty in deciding which orientation to use is evident in the *b* of *bushes,* the *z* of *lazy* and the *p* of *spoil* which were the three words dictated for the first line. The second line shows trouble with the *f* and *t* as described above. The child could spell both *transfer* and *suffer* orally without error. It may be noted here that in the second *f* of *suffer,* she has avoided the puzzle presented by the lower case forms by using a capital F. In the bottom line can be seen the tendency to backward progression and distorted order. In writing *green,* this girl produced *neer* before she saw her error and partially erased it—leaving, however, "ghosts" of the letters which could be traced for the illustration. Similarly, *of* was written first as *Fo,* again using the capital, and then changed to *oF*. The last word in this line was meant for *stop*.

A further fact of interest in the poor readers is the facility which some of them show in reading reversed or mirrored print. Printed material may be shown to a child so that he sees it in a mirror, or text may be produced in reverse on the typewriter by inserting a sheet of carbon paper face up, thus producing a mirrored copy on the back of the overlying paper, or better still, type can be secured from type-founders which give a mirrored imprint, which are called offset

Problems in Children

type, and test cards printed from these. In rare cases the skill of a child in reading these sinistrad words or sentences is better than his ability with material printed in the dextrad or ordinary direction, and this may extend to both speed and numbers of words correctly read. More commonly, however, the child requires a longer time to read the mirrored passage but very frequently shows a relative skill in this if the ratio of the time required for reading comparable paragraphs in both directions be taken and compared with that of normal readers of the same age, grade and intelligence. The data for determining this relative skill were published as part of the studies in the reading disability carried out in Iowa several years ago.

Occasionally the same factor of reversal which is to be seen in reading also causes trouble in arithmetic. The child may misread 12 as 21, for example, or may get into difficulty with the direction to be followed in carrying when adding, or in borrowing when subtracting. Compared with the number and length of the sequences of letters to be remembered in order to recognize words, however, those of arithmetic are simple and are usually quickly straightened out although the tendency to miswrite 12 as 21 is apt to persist after its recognition is secure, much as the tendency to miswrite a *b* or a *d* often remains long after the child can discriminate by eye between them. Usually the arithmetical processes do not make serious trouble for the children who are non-readers, if they have normal general intelligence, and they frequently present a striking contrast in their ability in handling numbers and their difficulty in mastering words. With those children who have spent several years in school without recognition of their reading disability or without adequate retraining, it is not unusual to find on standardized tests that the results in arithmetic are several school grades ahead of those in reading and spelling. As would be expected, however, the poor reader is seriously handicapped in understanding the directions on such tests and can often make comparatively little headway with the story or reasoning type of problem as contrasted with his ability in simple computation. To obtain a just estimate of the arithmetical ability it is obviously necessary to read the problems aloud to the child, and when this is done the prompt and accurate answers often demonstrate that an apparent difficulty with the problem type of examination rests in its reading requirements and not in the ability to handle the arithmetical concepts. We have encountered a few strephosymbolic children, with superior intelligence, who were failing in arithmetic as well as in reading in the upper grades, but this appeared to be directly attributable to poor teaching or to a demonstrable emotional factor in the situation and in every case in which special tutoring was provided for the arithmetic as well as for reading, the arithmetic responded quickly whereas the reading was found to require special methods and a much longer period of remedial training.

Spelling forms an almost insuperable obstacle to the strephosymbolic child. Since his memory of the word picture is not exact enough to serve as a basis for its recognition when *seen* again as in attempting to read, it is not surprising to find that the much more accurate recall needed for reproduction also fails, and in greater degree. With very severe cases and with untreated

Problems in Children

moderately severe cases observed during the first two or three years of school, there is usually no progress in either reading or spelling which can be measured by standardized tests. With cases of less severity and when proper treatment has been instituted, progress is made in both subjects but the ability to recognize words almost always outruns the ability to reproduce them correctly so that spelling as a rule lags considerably behind reading. Moreover, unless very careful attention by appropriate methods be given to spelling as well as to reading, the child may progress very little in the former. These children can often learn to spell words by rote auditory memory but this is apt to be very short lived, so that repeated drilling by spelling lists of words out loud often has very little permanent effect. Occasionally the rote memory will carry a considerable list of words for a time so that in some instances one finds the child able to spell all of the words of his current school grade but exceedingly defective in those of the earlier grades, long since forgotten. Errors may be of equal number and degree in both oral and written spelling or one may be harder than the other. When this is the case it is usually the written spelling which is the more difficult. The errors which are made in spelling are of many varieties but it is of interest to note that here also, distortions in the order of recall of the letters belonging in a word are outstanding and that among these are to be seen typical confusions between *b* and *d,* and *p* and *q,* as well as reversals of paired letters, syllables and whole words, such as are to be found in the reading errors. Not infrequently one encounters a child who gives no history of delay in acquisition of silent reading understanding

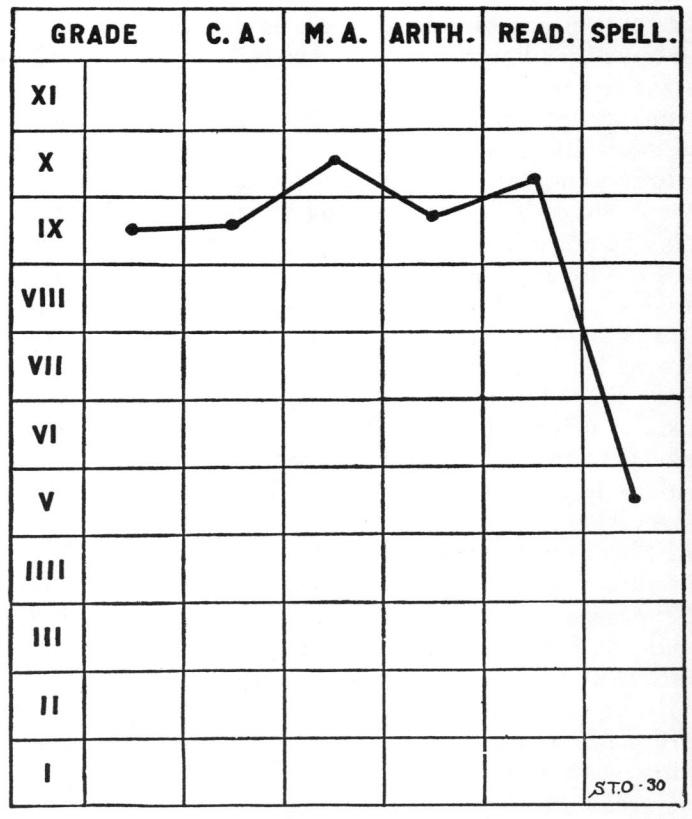

GRADE	C. A.	M. A.	ARITH.	READ.	SPELL.
XI					
X					
IX					
VIII					
VII					
VI					
V					
IIII					
III					
II					
I					

FIGURE 9. *Educational profile of a fourteen-year-old boy with a special spelling disability. C.A. indicates chronological age. M.A. indicates mental age.*

Problems in Children

but who does have great difficulty with spelling. Usually, in such cases, tests of *oral* reading capacity show many deficiencies in this technique and the character of the spelling errors suggests strongly that this disability rests on the same basis as does that which usually accompanies the severe reading disorder. Figure 9 shows the educational profile of a case of special disability in spelling. This was a boy who gave a history of a very slow start in learning to read although, as the profile demonstrates, he had finally gained a good skill in this. His oral reading was still poor as it is apt to be in the poor spellers. The headings in this figure are the same as those explained in connection with Figures 4, 5 and 6.

In extremely severe cases of strephosymbolia the visual recall of the details of the word may be so defective that unless the child has been taught the phonetic values of the letters, he is quite hopelessly at sea in spelling and some of his attempts produce the most bizarre results. The product may be so unlike the word attempted as to constitute a true neographism and a whole composition of such words presents a startling appearance. A classical example of this is a school composition offered as a description of the British Campaign of 1777 in the American Revolution which was handed in by a boy of sixteen years of age who had never learned to read. This is produced in facsimile in Figure 10. When this boy was permitted to dictate his compositions, he produced a creditable performance, showing that the ideas were there and also the words to express them, but when he attempted to write down what he had just dictated the same sort of errors appeared as are found in this composition. This

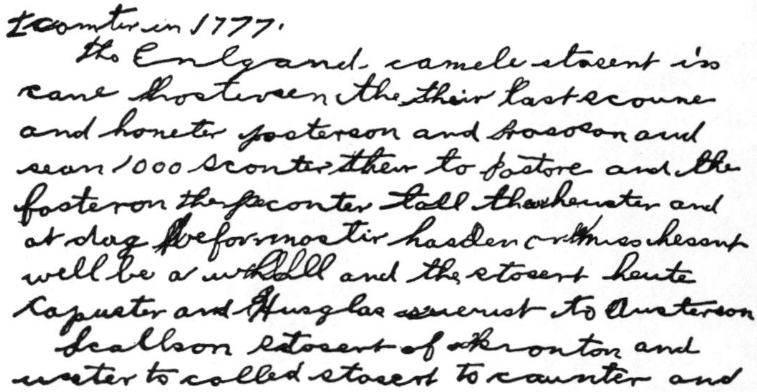

FIGURE 10. *Unintelligible neographisms produced by a sixteen-year-old boy with a severe reading disability. This material was submitted as a composition descriptive of the English campaign in 1777 in a high-school course in American History.*

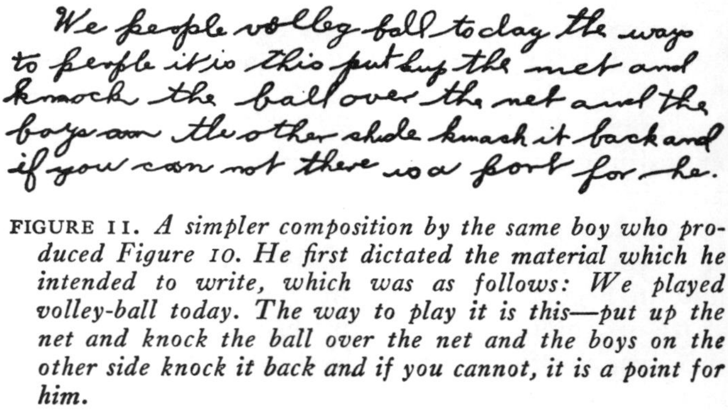

FIGURE 11. *A simpler composition by the same boy who produced Figure 10. He first dictated the material which he intended to write, which was as follows: We played volley-ball today. The way to play it is this—put up the net and knock the ball over the net and the boys on the other side knock it back and if you cannot, it is a point for him.*

Problems in Children

is shown in Figure 11. Thus it is apparent that the linkage or association between the component sounds of a word and the proper letters to represent them was as defective as was that between the letter and its proper sound, as shown by his complete inability to read any but a few familiar words and his utter helplessness with nonsense syllables. He was, however,

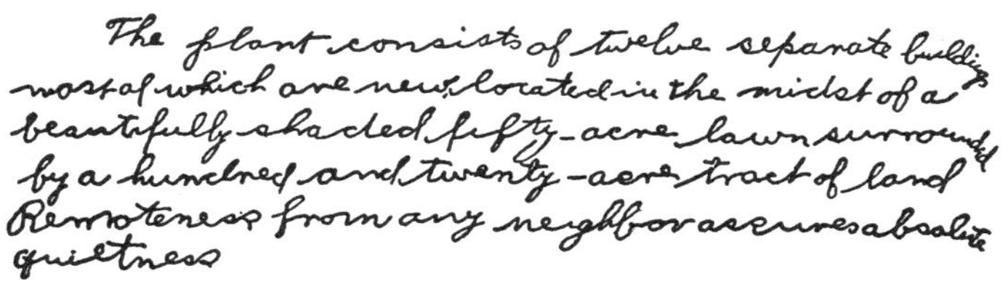

FIGURE 12. *Copying from print into script by the same boy who produced Figures 10 and 11. The marked contrast between copying and propositional work is seen by comparing this with Figures 10 and 11.*

able to copy from print into his own characteristic script in practically letter perfect form although he understood nothing of what he was writing. His copying is shown in Figure 12.

The handwriting of children with a reading disability is a variable. Not infrequently they show evidence of a much greater difficulty in acquiring printing or writing than would be expected from their dexterity in other manual skills, and hence fall clearly in the group of special writing disabilities which will be discussed later in this volume. Others, however, encounter no such selective obstacle and learn to write without undue difficulty.

Studies of laterality in the cases of developmental alexia have shown a very considerable number of crossed patterns between handedness and eyedness, as well as other forms of motor intergrading, but this is by no means without exception and we have encountered extreme cases of the reading disability in children who were right-sided as well as in those who were completely left-sided. Manual dexterity is variable in the group but often is quite highly developed. This is also true of general athletic skill and we find no motor problems consistently associated with the reading disability. Since developmental alexia is primarily a difficulty in recognition and hence falls in the category of sensory disorders, the problem of the child's handedness is of no importance from the standpoint of retraining unless there be a coexistent writing disability, speech defect, or apraxia. The presence among the reading disability cases, however, of a large number of children who show mixed or crossed motor patterns is considered suggestive evidence that as a group they belong among the intergrades, and this is borne out by the fact that the family history in by far the great majority of cases shows the presence of left-handedness in the stock and very often language disorders of one sort or another in other members of the family as well.

The milder cases of strephosymbolia gradually learn to read, but usually very poorly as compared with the accomplishment of others of their age and general intelligence. As they progress in school work, both the volume and the intricacy of the reading demands increase to the place where they surpass the child's ability, and academic progress may then be definitely

Problems in Children

blocked. Thus we meet these cases failing in the secondary schools and even in college through inability to read with sufficient speed to cover their assignments or through difficulty in understanding the material which they have studied because of misreading of words. Upon tests of silent reading comprehension these pupils occasionally come up to the norms for school children of their age but usually fall considerably below the expected achievement for their intelligence and general background. Silent reading, moreover, permits of skimming to grasp the general intent of a sentence or paragraph without the necessity of reading every word with understanding, and when the pupil is confronted with the much more precise task required by reading aloud many errors come to light and not infrequently some of these are of a nature to explain difficulties in understanding the content. Confusions of words with somewhat similar configurations and not too dissimilar meanings are frequent, as when *house* is read for *home, sugar* for *syrup,* etc. Reversals such as we see in the younger children are rare although they occur occasionally even among the college students and can sometimes be brought out by the use of compound nonsense syllables when they are not to be seen in reading meaningful words. Misreading or the omission of small words is common, and this often will completely change the meaning of the text. Not infrequently questions concerning the meanings of words which have been misread or mispronounced will disclose serious confusions between words which are roughly similar in appearance, and at times the problem of competence of auditory discrimination will arise as when words which sound somewhat alike are also confused. In one fourteen-year-old girl, for example, the word *phenomena* met in print was read as "fmonia" and when she was asked at a subsequent visit what was meant by "fmonia" she parried with the question, "Do you mean the liquid or the disease?" Obviously her interchange of *phenomena* and *pneumonia* was the result of their visual similarity while that of *pneumonia* and *ammonia* rested on their auditory likeness. From all of these she had constructed the neologism "fmonia" which might serve for any of the three. Comparable confusions are in some cases very numerous as, for example, when *deference* is read as *difference, laughter* as *loiter, flock* as *float, experiment* as *experience,* and *aggregation* as *exaggeration.* These and many others appeared in the oral reading of a fourteen-year-old boy with superior intelligence but with a residual strephosymbolia. At this age it is often impossible to say how much of such confusion results from faulty recall of the precise details of the printed word and from failure to learn its spelling and how much may represent a residuum of a complicating auditory word difficulty.

Among the older children—of late secondary school or college age—who give a history of a clear cut early reading disability, we have met several who have learned to read individual words accurately and who have acquired a good vocabulary but who have great difficulty in gaining the meaning from reading of long sentences or paragraphs. Not infrequently such a patient will be able to define accurately and without hesitation all the words in the material read and yet fail to grasp the significance of the sentences into which they are combined. The oral reading in such cases is apt to be a jerky, word by word procedure with very little of the emphasis demanded by major and dependent clauses, giving the impression that while each unit of the longer phrases and sentences is grasped, the grammatical sequence and hence comprehension are far from facile. These children complain of the time required to cover reading assignments with understanding and of the frequent need of rereading or even of more or less analyzing their required reading before being able to comprehend it thoroughly.

Spelling constitutes a major hurdle to children of this group. It is not uncommon to find their achievement in this subject lagging five or more grades behind their placement in school and their accomplishment in mathematics. Usually it is from one to several years below their silent reading ability but is apt to be much nearer the rating which they achieve in oral reading tests. Sometimes the words which make them the most trouble are the smaller words which they should have learned during their earlier years in school. Their errors are of the same general order as those of the younger children, notably misplacements and the choice of the wrong diphthongs or phonograms to represent a sound, showing their difficulty in the visual recall of the exact word picture. Reversals are not an outstanding feature but they are not uncommon. Often a misspelled word is recognized as such by the child with the remark, "I can see that it isn't right but I can't see what's wrong with it." Erasures and changes are frequent and many times a word that is correctly spelled upon the first attempt "looks wrong" to the child and he will add a few extra letters for good measure. As with the younger children, an occasional individual of this older group will show an extreme disability in spelling without the poor reading which more commonly accompanies it. No essential difference has been found in the type of errors made by these two groups of bad spellers. When the reading is not involved, there will be no difficulty, of course, in learning from books, but these children are heavily penalized in their written work because of their poor spelling, which may actually prevent their papers from being accepted, no matter how excellent they be in other respects.

    These older children with a history of serious delay in learning to read while in the lower grades usually encounter trouble again when they take up the study of foreign languages. With many of them the ability to learn by ear is sufficiently well developed so that they have little or no trouble learning to converse in French or German, but the reading, writing, spelling and formal grammar that usually form so large a part of the instruction in preparatory school and college courses offer much the same sort of obstacles which the child met when he was first assigned similar tasks in learning English. Often when a new language is begun the first step is that of teaching the characteristic phonetic values of the letters of the alphabet in that tongue, and this occasionally makes the learning in the new language easier than might otherwise have been true, but by and large the borderline strephosymbolic is not a good prospect for the learning of new languages and his path is apt to be thorny particularly if, as sometimes is the case, he is at work in several of these new subjects at once.

    Among the children of secondary school age who have been studied because of scholastic failures which

Problems in Children

were out of harmony with their general promise and their accomplishments in other than linguistic fields, we have met some with a degree of difficulty on the expressive side which has seemed very much more severe than would be expected from their apparent understanding. In a few this has involved both spoken and written expression but in the majority it has been much more prominent in writing. The poor spellers as a group are usually also poor in grammar, punctuation, sentence structure, etc., and occasionally this is so severe and so at variance with the understanding of printed material, with the general intelligence and maturing judgment of the individual, as to raise the question as to whether or not it may constitute a specific disorder in verbal expression comparable to acquired agrammatism. When severe, the condition serves as a decisive handicap in written examinations, and when it interferes with both oral and written expression the chance of a satisfactory adjustment in either academic or social activities is distinctly limited. Such cases form one of the more recent extensions of our studies in the language delays, and methods for a satisfactory approach to their diagnosis are still in a highly experimental stage, but they are a group of great interest and no little challenge.

The children with a specific reading disability are almost never interested in reading for pastime. Their whole tendency is to turn to athletics or mechanics or social activities as an outlet and it is not uncommon to find a child almost up to college age who has read practically nothing except those books which have been required in the school courses. Indeed, one of our college patients won a prize in a book-review contest when in high school by presenting a clever theme entitled "I Have Never Read A Book"! Naturally the restricted intake through lack of reading over a long period strikingly limits the store of words available for expression. The occasional individual may compensate to some degree for this by facility in the auditory field and so develop a good speaking vocabulary, but usually both spoken and written vocabularies are poor, and written compositions and examinations on which so much of academic progress depends fall far below the pupil's probable potentialities had his training from the beginning been suited to his needs. Long experience with indifferent academic success or failure in spite of hard effort may eventually dull the zest for learning even in the most conscientious pupil, and we find many of these older students apparently acquiescent to their status as failures or near failures in each succeeding class, although sometimes their ambition does withstand their discouraging experiences and they persist in the conviction that they will master their difficulties in time and often optimistically present plans to study law or medicine although at the age of nineteen or twenty they are still deficient in most of their high school work. Their rating on intelligence and scholastic aptitude tests, which are usually composed largely of linguistic material, frequently drops below that obtained in earlier examinations but often is found to be higher than their output in the classroom would lead one to expect. It is frequently hard to determine in these older cases how much of the current difficulty is due to residuals of strephosymbolia and how much to poor early training. Typical reading troubles are often reported by the parents to

Problems in Children

have been suspected by them in early school years but to have been either overlooked or underestimated by the school, or left uncorrected for one reason or another. In other cases there is a history of some extra help having been given to the child by various teachers in the lower grades and of considerable repetitive tutoring and intensive cramming of special subjects during vacations after the pupil has advanced into the secondary schools, but with no recognition of the fact that a fundamental language difficulty may underlie failures in such subjects as history and French, for example.

The presence of residuals of an old reading disability, expressing themselves in slow and inaccurate oral reading, considerable difficulty in grasping the meaning of even moderately complex material read silently and difficulty with spelling and written expression, often brings up the question of how far advanced academic education will be really profitable. Most parents want their children to finish high school or preparatory school and to make at least an attempt at college. The rigidity of college entrance examinations together with the foreign languages which are required for admission often serve to prevent such a student from going to one of the larger colleges and, unfortunately, the smaller colleges are not infrequently those which have clung most closely to the classical tradition and whose curriculum therefore is heavily laden with languages, while the sciences, in which the pupil would have the best chance of success, are not so freely available. In some cases, the experimental, so-called progressive colleges have admitted these students without the usual entrance requirements in English or foreign languages, but here independent and creative work is highly

98   Reading, Writing and Speech

stressed and the boy or girl who is unfamiliar with books, who cannot cover a large amount of collateral reading and who is inept in written expression, is again faced with obstacles which are often insurmountable. In two such cases where the students' interests were primarily in drama, their difficulty in oral reading prevented them from successful competition in the tryouts for parts in dramatic productions. When the language problem is recognized for the first time at the high school age, there has often accrued so great a deficit in familiarity with words through lack of reading, which may in turn have seriously interfered with the development of understanding, that the question must often be raised as to whether this can be overcome by even the most careful retraining program in time to prepare the pupil for college before he is far past the usual age for it, and whether or not the same time spent in vocational training or on a job would not in the long run put him much further ahead than an effort at collegiate education.

To summarize briefly the clinical picture of strephosymbolia we may say that we are here confronted with a group of children presenting all degrees of difficulty in learning to recall a printed or written word with sufficient accuracy to recognize it (reading) or to reproduce it (spelling). While some children who show this syndrome may also exhibit concurrent disorders in other fields of language as, for example, in learning to write or in an adequate mastery of spoken language, yet many of them show no such complications and the most searching examinations reveal no other deviations in the function of the brain except this difficulty with the recall of word pictures, and hence they are much

Problems in Children

more selective than the "purest" of cases of alexia in the adult in which a certain measure of interference with other functions than that of reading is always to be observed if the examining methods be exhaustive enough. In this respect developmental alexia is unique and may indeed in time come to be recognized as a pure syndrome which will warrant further study for a better understanding of the acquired condition as well as for its own inherent interest and its great practical value to education.

2. *Developmental Agraphia (Special Writing Disability)*

Another group of children find special difficulty in learning to write. This may, as has been mentioned, coexist with the reading disability and the associated trouble with spelling, but the writing disability is also encountered not infrequently as an isolated developmental disorder. This special difficulty in learning to write may exhibit itself in one of two ways. In the first, the child may be able to form letters well and produce a neat and acceptable writing from a qualitative standpoint, but the process may be so slow as to constitute a definite obstacle to school advancement. An example of this type is the case of a boy who was quite unable to finish more than half of any class assignment requiring writing although what he did complete was neatly and accurately done. He was quite regularly receiving grades of about 50% on his written work, which represented an almost perfect mark for the amount of ground which he had been able to cover in the time allowed for each examination. Figure 13 shows the educational profile of such a case. This was

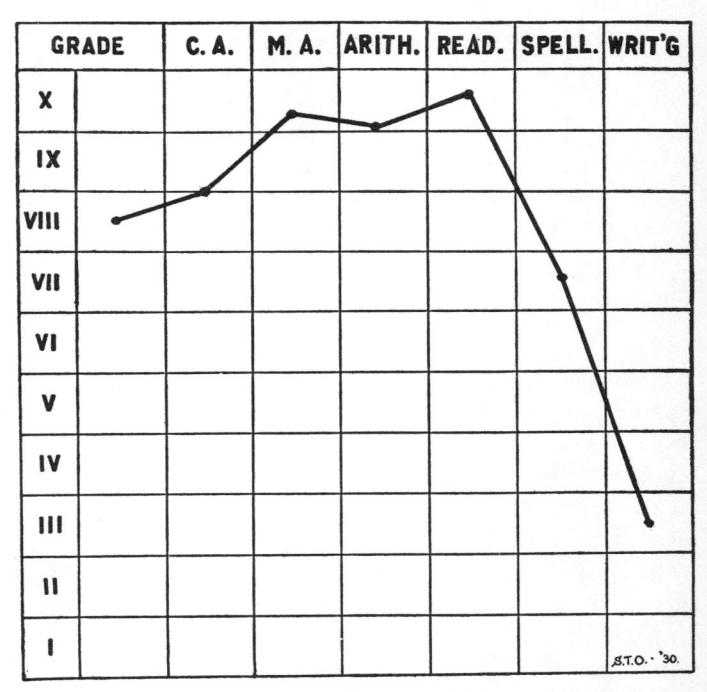

GRADE	C. A.	M. A.	ARITH.	READ.	SPELL.	WRIT'G
X						
IX						
VIII						
VII						
VI						
V						
IV						
III						
II						
I						

FIGURE 13. *Educational profile of a fifteen-year-old shifted left-handed boy with a marked special writing disability. The abbreviations are the same as those in preceding profiles.*

a fifteen-year-old left-handed boy who was taught to write with his right hand and, while the product was of fair quality, he was able to produce while copying only the number of letters per minute that are to be expected of an eight-year-old as measured by the Ayres Handwriting Scale. The second type of this disability is that in which the quality of the writing suffers. In speed, these latter children are variable; some of them are slow, as well as poor writers, while others achieve a good speed but the quality of their product is far from acceptable and often quite illegible.

In many cases of this difficulty there is a history of a shift from the left to the right hand in early infancy, or an enforced training of the right hand for writing in spite of a strong preference for the left as exhibited in all spontaneously acquired skills. These shifted sinistrals seem a little more apt to fall into the group of slow writers rather than poor writers, although there is no consistency in this. Figure 14 shows an example of the handwriting of a boy of this group. His left-handedness was recognized and accepted in everything except eating at the table and writing, where a right-handed pattern had been enforced. The upper part of the illustration gives inherent evidence of the difficulty he was finding in acquiring an acceptable writing skill while the lower part shows the results after he had been taught to write with his naturally superior hand. In this instance the training of the left hand for writing was not begun until the boy was fifteen years old. Sometimes when right-hand training of a natural sinistral has been instituted very early, the usages acquired through a number of years of such training may effectively hide the natural bent, and such cases of "masked" left-handedness can often be recognized only by the use of motor tests. Figure 15 shows the handwriting of such a case. Here the boy's tendency to use his left hand had been noted in infancy and he had been purposely trained to use the right. At the time of his examination at the age of eleven, he was considered

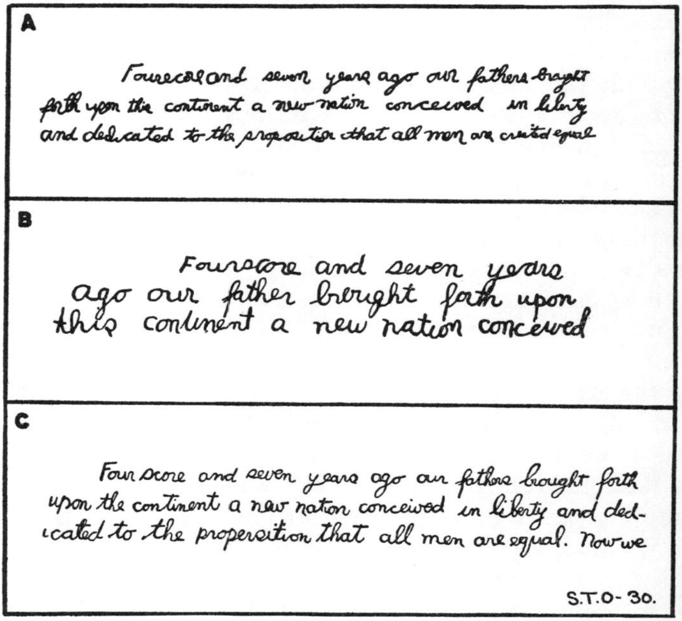

> **A**
> Fourscore and seven years ago our fathers brought forth upon the continent a new nation conceived in liberty and dedicated to the proposition that all men are created equal
>
> **B**
> Fourscore and seven years ago our father brought forth upon this continent a new nation conceived
>
> **C**
> Fourscore and seven years ago our fathers brought forth upon the continent a new nation conceived in liberty and dedicated to the proposition that all men are equal. Now we
>
> S.T.O-30.

FIGURE 14. *Writing of the same boy whose profile is shown in Figure 13. At A is an example of his right-hand writing when first examined. B shows the product of his left hand at the same time. It was then only one-half as fast as the right. At C is shown the effect of two months' training of the left hand for writing. In this time it had acquired the same speed as the right hand.*

by his parents, by his teachers and even by himself to be right-handed, but motor tests showed a much better latent skill in the left and he was consequently shifted to that hand in all his activities including writing. The upper half of the illustration shows a fair sample of

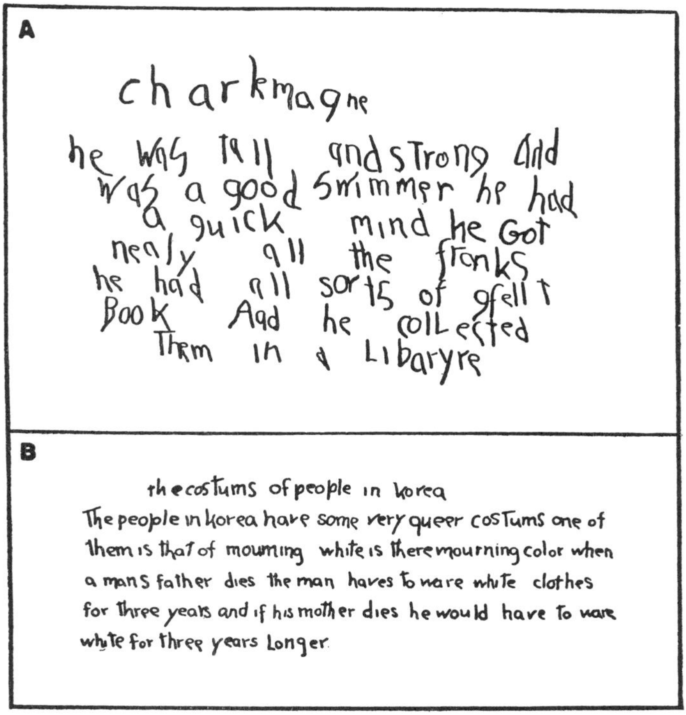

> **A**
>
> charkmagne
> he was ill and strong and
> was a good swimmer he had
> a quick mind he Got
> nealy all the fronks
> he had all sorts of gell t
> Book Aad he collected
> Them in a Libaryre
>
> **B**
>
> the costums of people in korea
> The people in korea have some very queer costums one of
> them is that of mourning white is there mourning color when
> a mans father dies the man haves to ware white clothes
> for three years and if his mother dies he would have to ware
> white for three years longer.

FIGURE 15. *Special writing disability in a "masked left-hander," eleven years of age. At A is shown the product of his right hand after five years of intensive training while B shows his left-hand writing one year later.*

his writing after five years in school. The lower half shows the product with his left hand one year later.

It is not infrequent to find that a left-handed child,

104   Reading, Writing and Speech

when he first starts to write, produces everything in the mirrored or sinistrad form, and indeed there is some reason to believe that this is the natural or spontaneous direction for the left-handed. Figure 16 is an

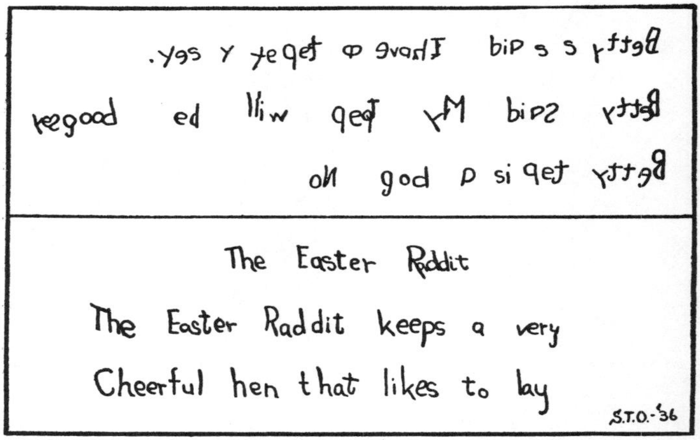

>>>
Betty gets a dad. No.
Betty said My dad will be good.
Betty gets a dad. Thank you very much.

The Easter Raddit
The Easter Raddit keeps a very
Cheerful hen that likes to lay   S.T.O.-'36
<<<

FIGURE 16. *Writing of a left-handed boy. At the top is his spontaneous mirror-writing produced during his first year in school. Below is his product one year later when everything except the confusing b's and d's had been reoriented. Both examples were produced with his left hand.*

excellent example of this. At the top of the figure is shown the product of a six-year-old left-handed boy writing with his left hand and showing almost complete sinistrad reversal. It may be noted that in the fifth word—the article *a*—he was in some confusion and produced a doubled letter, while in the next word, which is "pet," he has spelled it both ways as t-e-p-e-t and in the last word on that line he has reversed his direction. The lower part of the figure shows his writing—still with the left hand—one year later when dextrad progress had been acquired and dextrad orientation in all the letters except the *b*'s in "rabbit." In addition, however, to the fact that the left-handed child probably has to acquire an orientation and progress opposite to that which would be most facile for him, he is all too frequently met by another difficulty in that the paper is put before him in the same position in which it would be placed for a right-handed child, which forces the left-hander to adopt the cramped and awkward position so often to be seen. The proper position to prevent this trouble will be discussed later in this volume.

In addition to the frank left-handers and those whose left-hand tendency has been masked by early training of the right, we have seen a number of patients who were indifferent in their handedness and who had less than the average skill in finer movements of the hands and fingers of either side and whose poor writing seemed to rest on this basis. In some of these the difficulty extended to the learning of any new manual manipulation and was extreme enough to be likened to an apraxia; in others it was sharply restricted to the movements of writing and it was among these latter that two interesting clinical observations were made. In one girl of eleven it was possible to demonstrate a high degree of dexterity in the finer movements of the fingers and the hand for a wide variety of activities, including the use of the pencil for drawing. She was able to draw each letter, singly, with ease and nicety, but the process of blending the letters into

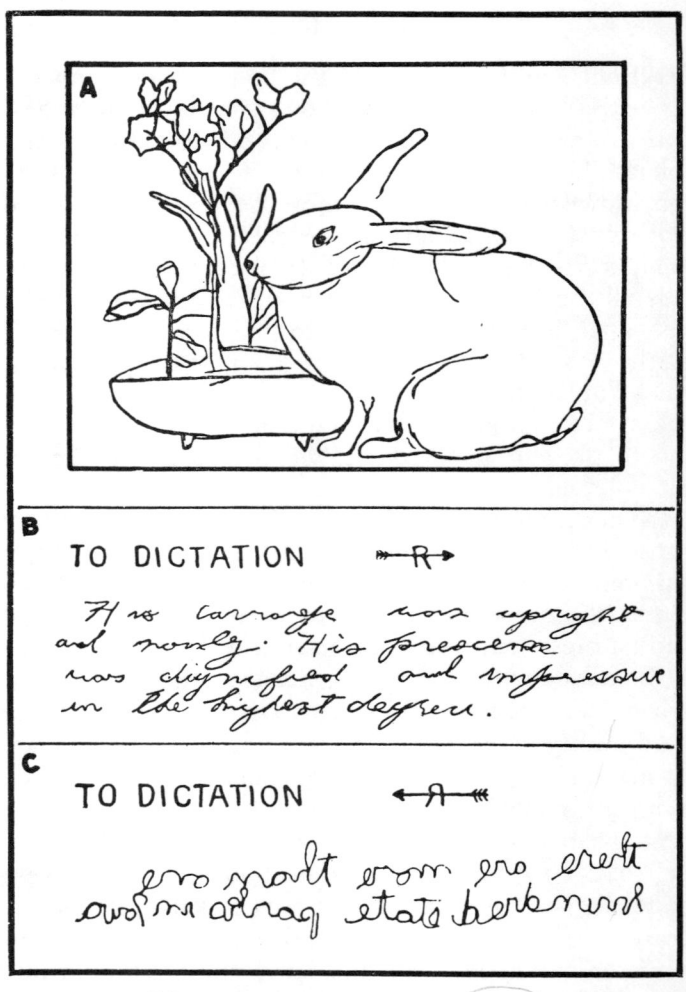

FIGURE 17. *Mirror-writing ability in an eleven-year-old girl who had great difficulty in learning to write in the dextrad direction. A further explanation of this figure is given in the text.*

Problems in Children 107

words with anything like acceptable speed for her age had resisted years of hard work on the part of both herself and her teachers. In the course of a routine examination of her skills, however, it was found that while she could not write successfully in the dextrad or ordinary direction with the right hand and showed no skill in writing in either direction with the left, yet she could, without practice, produce quite a respectable product with her right hand if written in the sinistrad or mirrored form. Figure 17 shows this girl's product. At A in the illustration is shown a sketch made from objects in her home which indicates a clever use of the pencil. At B is a sample of her usual writing in the dextrad form. At C is shown a part of her first attempt at mirror writing. If the reader will examine this before a mirror, its quality as compared with the dextrad will be immediately seen. Not only, however, was the quality good, but writing in this direction was also a much more facile procedure. Another patient who showed this symptom in striking form was a twenty-one-year-old medical student who had never been able to learn to write acceptably in the ordinary direction. With plenty of time and in simple material he could write so that it could be deciphered, but under pressure for time, as in taking notes in college, or when the propositional element was marked, as in answering examination questions, his writing was not only illegible to others but he himself could not read it. He was right-handed and possessed of at least the average manual dexterity as evinced in the dissecting room and in laboratory manipulations. Again, in this case, no latent writing skills were found in the left hand, but

108 Reading, Writing and Speech

from the very first trial he was able to produce a legible and really quite creditable script in the mirrored form with his right hand. Figure 18 shows at the top a sample of his writing to dictation which is more legible than the average of his propositional efforts, and below, a sample of his mirror writing produced within a

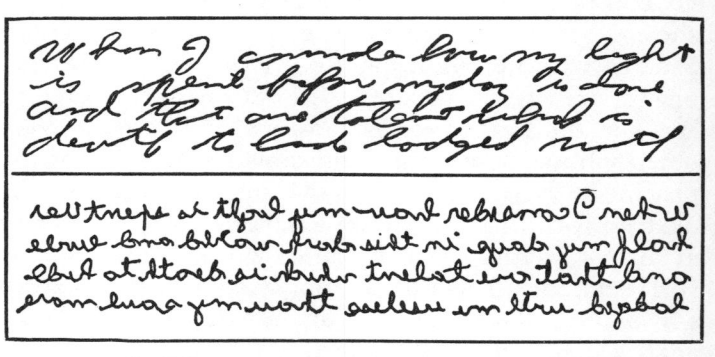

FIGURE 18. *Mirror-writing with the right hand produced by a 21-year-old student with a marked specific writing disability. Further explanation is given in the text.*

week after his first introduction to this procedure. Again, if the reader will examine the lower part of this illustration with a mirror, the contrast between the product in the two directions will be strikingly apparent. A number of others of our specific writing disability cases have shown this symptom in varying degree of perfection, but so far it has not appeared in those cases in whom motor skills were clearly below average on both sides. The capacity to write in the sinistrad form is not an unusual accomplishment and one occasionally meets an individual who can write in either direction

Problems in Children

with either hand with almost equal skill. Figure 19 shows an example of this. The interest in the mirrored writing in the special disability cases, however, rests not so much on the presence of this skill as the fact that it was acquired without training and without practice during the long period when the patient was strug-

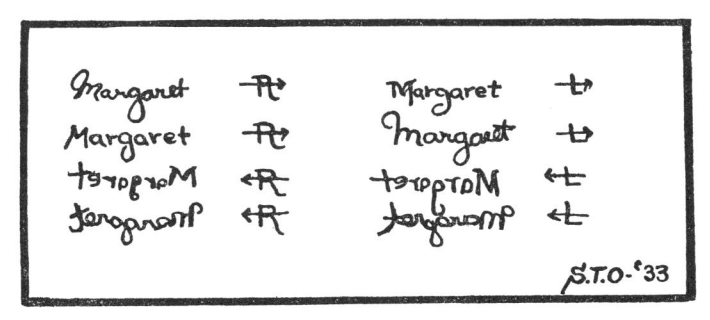

FIGURE 19. *Skillful writing in either direction and with either hand. The initials indicate the hand used and the arrows show the direction of writing.*

gling unsuccessfully to acquire the dextrad or ordinary form of progress. This fact is worthy of especial note.

A second interesting fact observed in certain children who were having great difficulty in learning to write was the capacity to produce a somewhat better formed and more regular hand while their eyes were directed away from the paper or while they were blindfolded than while they were watching the writing hand. Figure 20 gives a fair example of this. Our attention was directed to the possible confusing element brought in by current visual impressions by a study in the Language Research Laboratory of the Neurological Institute of a case of aphasia following a fracture of the skull and damage to the brain. This patient was entirely unsuccessful in copying various geometric figures on the board while looking at them but could study such a design for a moment, close his eyes and then produce a highly satisfactory replica.

The special writing disability in those cases which

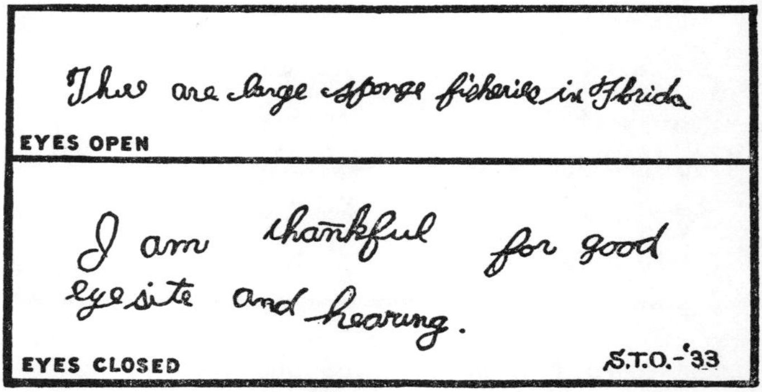

> **EYES OPEN**
> *There are large sponge fisheries in Florida*
>
> **EYES CLOSED**
> *I am thankful for good eyesite and hearing.*   S.T.O.-'33

FIGURE 20. *Contrast between writing while watching paper and while blindfolded, produced by a thirteen-year-old boy.*

are not the result of faulty training, enforced shift of handedness, or marked motor intergrading, and which is not associated with reading or spelling disability, again exemplifies, even more clearly than does strephosymbolia, that the developmental disorders of language in children may exist in much purer form than do the comparable syndromes resulting from brain damage in the adult since *acquired* motor agraphia without other complicating disorders (notably of speech) is so rare that many authors deny its existence as an entity.

3. Developmental Word Deafness

There are cases described in the medical literature under the name of congenital word deafness but they are few enough to have been looked upon heretofore as decided rarities. The presenting symptom in these cases is a difficulty in recognition of the spoken word and a consequent delay and distortion of speech, but with normal hearing. As with the term word blindness, "word deafness" is misleading since it can be clearly shown that typical cases of this nature have normal hearing throughout the whole of the audible range and can hear the word accurately but do not understand it.

In these children as in adults with acquired word deafness, the audiometer gives an entirely normal picture. There is, moreover, no difficulty with the understanding of sounds of the environment—bells, whistles, etc.—other than words, and this condition forms therefore a very close analogy in the auditory field to strephosymbolia in the visual, in that there is no trouble with reception nor is there any difficulty with the elaboration of sensation until the word level is reached, but here the sharply defined disorder appears. When word deafness is suspected, careful tests of hearing are of utmost importance. With older children a test of the complete audible range on any standard audiometer is possible.

In very young or distractible children such tests are of course out of the question, and we must depend on our observations of their reactions to tuning forks, music and other sounds, and here a real difficulty enters through the presence of a condition which is apparently that of auditory inattention. Such youngsters at times react to various sounds and at other times pay no attention whatsoever to sounds of even greater intensity, and this is particularly true of spoken words. With the normal growing child, during his period of acquisition of word understanding and of speech, we expect a fairly close attention to words which are spoken to him, and even very active young children usually can be interested in nursery rhymes or stories read aloud to them. Apparently, however, in the children of the group which we are now discussing, the spoken word does not serve to attract attention freely. If the spoken word carries no meaning, it is easy to see why the child does not react to it. Indeed the sounds of speech around him would be disregarded as adults disregard the sounds of traffic or other adventitious noises of the environment. Occasionally this factor is so striking that a real question arises in the minds of the parents and others who are working with the child as to whether or not a true deafness is present.

True deafness, whether peripheral or central, does not belong in the category of disorders which we are discussing here. It forms a special and well developed field of study with its own methods of treatment, and such cases may therefore be excluded from our discussion. Audiometer tests, however, occasionally bring to light a special form of partial deafness which must be carefully differentiated from word deafness. This is the so-called high frequency deafness in which hearing is normal or nearly so for all pitches of the audible range except a few. The term "high frequency deafness" is not quite exact since occasionally lessened acuity may be found for only the lower pitches, as for

Problems in Children

example in bass deafness, and possibly the term "regional deafness," suggesting a reduced acuity in one region of the audible range, would better describe the condition. However, the higher frequencies are involved more commonly than the lower and the term high frequency deafness has already acquired wide usage. When such partial deafness involves those notes produced by vibration rates between 512 and 2048 double vibrations per second, which fall in the range required for spoken language, some difficulty with understanding may be encountered because the child cannot hear all of the sound units in a word. More commonly, however, enough sounds are caught to permit the understanding to develop with little or no serious interference, but defects appear in the child's speech. Generally, as shown by the audiometer curve, the hearing acuity drops sharply as the higher pitch ranges are reached and the defect in learning to speak is characterized by the elision particularly of those sounds which in themselves are high pitched, such as *s, f, th,* etc. Differentiation of the short sounds of the vowels *a, e, i* and *u* where the differences lie largely in the high-pitched overtones is also apt to be very defective. Children with this difficulty learn without instruction to cultivate a visual aid to understanding by watching the lips of the speaker and sometimes become quite proficient as lip readers. This reinforcement of hearing by watching the speaker is probably far more extensive in normal individuals than we usually appreciate since we all are apt to make use of it when listening intently to a voice which is faint or when in the presence of considerable noise. Advantage may be taken of this fact in examining children who have a speech disorder in which high frequency deafness is suspected, by having them echo after the examiner non-familiar material such as nonsense syllables, first while facing the examiner and watching his lips and then with their backs turned. Very often there is striking contrast between their capacity to echo the material under these two conditions. When a child is old enough to be given the audiometer test there is no difficulty whatsoever in the diagnosis of this condition. Before that, it is sometimes very hard indeed to say how much of a true regional deafness exists, how much word deafness, and how much a habit of auditory inattention. Figure 21 shows the audiogram of a typical case of high frequency deafness. The presenting symptom in this case was that of a speech defect rather than understanding. It will be noted that hearing is normal for notes up to 128 double vibrations per second. At 256 there is a slight loss in acuity while between 512 and 2048, which is the range used in speech, there is enough reduction to constitute a 50% loss as calculated by the Western Electric Audiometer scale.

Verbal understanding forms so large a factor in the acquisition of concepts and hence in the development of the intellect that anything interfering with the registration of words and their subsequent recall will of course sharply limit the mental development, and an, as yet, unanswerable question arises when we attempt to differentiate developmental word deafness, in its severe forms, from general intellectual defect. If a child is really deaf and is recognized as such, he can by appropriate methods be taught concepts and his intellect will continue to develop. When, however, the

Problems in Children

child obviously can hear, such methods will not be employed and if he does not learn the names of objects and concepts of his environment he may fail to develop

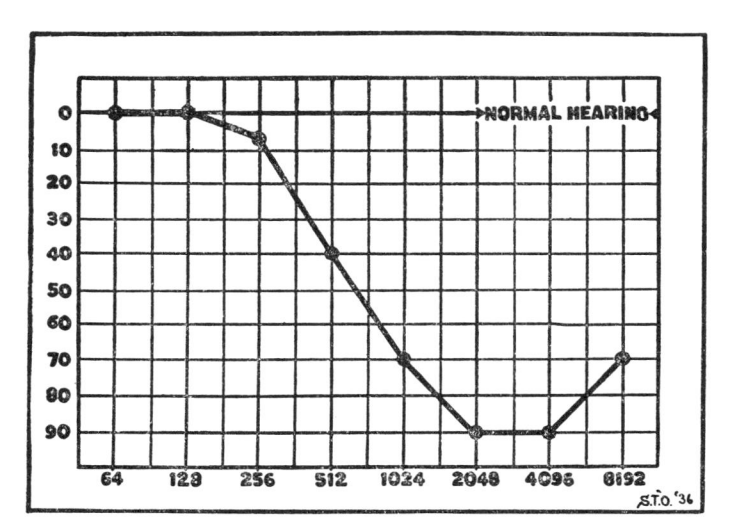

FIGURE 21. *Audiogram in a case of regional deafness of the high frequency type. The numbers in the vertical column at the left indicate sensation units. The numbers below indicate pitch as represented in double vibrations per second. The dots on the heavy line show the loss in hearing units for each pitch as found in this particular patient. The critical zone for speech lies between 512 and 2048 d.v. per sec.*

mentally and become truly feebleminded by deprivation. Our studies of this group are as yet rather few but have led us to believe that word deafness may be at the root of many cases which are now classed as feebleminded and may also be the basis of the failure to develop speech in some of the so-called hearing mutes in institutions for the deaf and dumb. Minor degrees of this sort of a difficulty shown in a marked tendency to misuse words through confusion with those of somewhat similar sound are to be seen on every hand. Typical of course is Mrs. Malaprop. Traces of word confusions like those seen in developmental word deafness are not infrequent in cases of the reading disability, as was indicated in the discussion of that condition.

In the majority of those cases where we believe this form of disorder to underlie a lack of normal language development and which were seen as young children, there has been a marked overactivity. The child, while inattentive to speech, is by no means inert but seems bent on investigating the environment to the best of his ability by vision, by touch, and at times even by smell. While speech is usually greatly delayed in its appearance, it does evolve slowly and at this stage there is a marked tendency to a prolonged period of echolalia and a prolix use of the small and often defective vocabulary which is available. In this there is an interesting parallel to the verbosity and paraphasia of the sensory aphasics in adult life. As these children grow older a variable degree of understanding of spoken words is attained, and here again it is noteworthy as in the case of the reading disabilities that the ability to understand individual words often far outruns the capacity to grasp the meaning of equally simple words when combined into sentences, particularly if the sentence be long or if the form of its presentation be somewhat unusual. The rate of intake of meanings is slow, as shown by the much better ability to understand it the speech delivery be deliberate and the words carefully enunciated. Often one simple command will be carried out promptly and correctly, while if a series of equally simple tasks be requested only one will be attempted and even that may end in failure. The verbal output of these older cases is marked by many errors both of pronunciation and of grammar. Omissions of some of the sounds of the word are very frequent. As examples of this may be quoted "spense" for "expense," "minds" for "reminds," "pose" for "suppose," "irresing" for "interesting" and even such extreme contractions as "flushey" for "flying ship." Parts of words may be distinctly distorted by the substitution of other sounds, as in "astinkly" for "distinctly," "repeller" for "propeller," "atween" for "between" and "ensify" for "emphasize." Confusions of properly enunciated words also appear as when "destruction" is used for "construction," "disaffection" for "defective" and "disgusting" for "discussing." There is also a tendency to drop out words from common phrases as when "quite a many people" is used for "quite a good many people" and "all sudden" for "all of a sudden." True neologisms also may appear, such as "ardless" used for "astronomer" and "phiägēs" for "physiologists." The varying forms of verbs seem to be especially difficult, leading to such expressions as "I have spoking," "They did all they can" and "thinking about to use" (using). Most of the examples of errors given here were from the speech of an extremely interesting boy of eighteen with normal hearing throughout the whole range as tested by the audiometer, normal understanding of sounds other than those of speech and normal appreciation of intensity, pitch and rhythm as shown by the Seashore musical appreciation tests, but a striking difficulty in both the receptive and reproductive functions when dealing with the spoken word.

Most of the children whom we have studied and whom we believe to belong in this category of developmental word deafness have given a history of marked delay in the time of development of speech and a striking lack of preferential choice of a master hand, and on testing have shown a definite "motor intergrading." The majority of those who were old enough to have made any efforts at reading have shown serious confusions of the strephosymbolic type when they encountered this subject. History of left-handedness or of some form of special language disability has been present in the families of most of these cases.

4. *Developmental Motor Aphasia (Motor Speech Delay)*

A fourth group of cases of developmental disorder in which we have been interested is that of children who are very slow in the development of speech and who usually show marked disorder in their speech as it develops but who have, in contrast to the word deafness cases, a good understanding of the spoken word. Their attention is usually quickly caught when they are spoken to and they often will listen carefully to what is said to them although they are somewhat more apt to be interested in doing things than in listening. They do not, however, show the striking degree of auditory inattention which is present in the word deafness cases, and would not be apt to be confused with deaf children. They use their hands freely in pointing to objects to obtain their desires but we have never seen any indication of the development of true symbolic gestures as in a sign language. They make efforts at verbalization in which they have a varying degree of success. In one four-year-old boy who probably belongs to this type there were no consonantal sounds at all in his attempts at propositional speech. He could echo quite a number of consonants after the examiner as separate phonetic units but could not use them either as blends with vowels in echoing or in his own efforts to talk. These children usually recognize their own speech errors to some extent and will not accept as correct a word pronounced by the examiner as they have given it, and this sometimes forms a diagnostic point of some value since it is in sharp contrast to the situation in the word deaf cases. Most of the children in this group are late in beginning to talk and likewise late in developing a preference for either the right or the left hand, and by the motor tests they usually show marked intergrading. In a few of our cases, history has been obtained of an abrupt onset of mutism after speech had started to develop, coinciding in time with efforts to train the child away from the preferred left hand. In one small boy such training efforts were accompanied by the development of a jargon which could not be understood at all but which cleared up strikingly as soon as he was allowed to use his left hand freely again in all of his activities.

These children with good understanding of the spoken word, but with little or no speech of their own, would seem to be closely analogous to cases of motor aphasia as seen in the adult. Milder cases apparently clear up spontaneously and such instances may be the source of the advice so frequently given to parents by their friends, "Let him alone and he will grow out of it." When speech is spontaneously acquired in these children, its development is apt to be very rapid, but a certain measure of speech defect often persists in the form of a lisp or a defective *r* or other infantilisms, and in several of our cases stuttering has appeared from the beginning of speech. Moreover, many of the child's early social adaptations will be seriously interfered with if he cannot talk freely with other children of his age. He is apt to be over-protected in the home because of his disability and often exhibits a marked emotional over-reaction to his feeling of frustration on vainly attempting to make himself understood, so that early speech training, which has given great promise in this type, would seem to be definitely indicated.

5. *Developmental Apraxia* (*Abnormal Clumsiness*)

The fifth group of cases to be discussed is that of developmental apraxia (congenital apraxia). The recognition of this type of individual goes back at least to Galen who spoke of some children as being "ambilevous," that is, doubly left-handed. Except for the unjustified implication as to the general unskillfulness of left-handers, this characterization fits the situation well. These children seem to be equipped with a lack of skill on both sides comparable to that of the left hand in a strongly right-handed person. The inability in this condition is for the carrying out of any complex trained movements whether they be of hand, foot, or body, and the question might be raised as to why this

Problems in Children

syndrome is included in a description of the developmental language delays. Two considerations have led to such inclusion. First, an acquired apraxia may result in the adult from a unilateral brain lesion, providing that lesion affect the dominant hemisphere, thus placing the control of highly skilled movements in the same group physiologically as the various language functions; and second, the difficulty of learning complex movements which characterizes the apraxias may extend to the motor patterns of both speech and writing as well as to the movements of the body and the extremities, and hence lead to specific language disorders in the motor or expressive field.

As stated above, there is a notable absence of skills on either side in these children and usually in spite of extended training there is a strong suggestion of a very close balance between the two hands. Motor tests often also show an amphiocularity or a lack of ability in monocular sighting by either eye. Such children are often somewhat delayed in learning even the simpler movements such as walking and running, and have great difficulty in learning to use their hands and to copy motions shown to them. They are slow in learning to dress themselves and are clumsy in their attempts to button their clothes, tie their shoes, handle a spoon, and in other simple tasks. One such boy recently studied had been slow in learning to walk and was awkward in his gait. He had mastered with some effort the riding of a three-wheel velocipede but the bicycle proved too much for him. Roller skating was likewise impossible for him as was baseball and almost all of the games of boyhood. In his case, his difficulty in learning motor patterns extended also to speech and writing. His speech was clipped and slurred, and although he could make all the sounds necessary for most words, his ability to blend them into a word and to use them properly in speech was very poor. In writing, neither hand had very much to recommend it and much effort over several years had failed to produce an acceptable penmanship. Although twelve years of age and equipped with normal intelligence, his motor patterns, on either side, were those of a much younger child and showed a marked intergrading.

6. *Stuttering in Childhood*

The last condition which we will discuss is that of stuttering. When encountered in the adult, stuttering has accumulated so great an emotional overlay that the problem of its genesis and treatment is much confused. This is a natural result of the experience of the individual who had been blocked, by reason of his impediment, from free social intercourse and who has very often indeed accumulated a heavy load of inferiority and a fear of speaking. In by far the great majority of stutterers, however, the difficulty with their speech began in childhood, and at the time of onset of stuttering, the picture is very different from that seen in the adult. The emotional and personality factors which are so striking later and which have led many observers to classify all stutterers as neurotics, are notably absent in childhood. Many early stutterers when seen within the first year of their difficulty show no demonstrable deviation in the emotional sphere and present no history of environmental or psychological difficulties which seem at all adequate to explain the

Problems in Children

disorder. For this reason and since this volume deals largely with the developmental period of language, attention will be given here only to the phenomena of stuttering as they are seen in early childhood.

It may be wise to recapitulate briefly here some of the neurological characteristics of the stuttering episode. Two types of muscular spasm are to be observed, a tonic contraction of the muscles which results in a complete block of speech and which is sometimes called stammering, and the clonic or repetitive spasm which gives rise to the typical stutter. There seems no valid reason to attempt to separate these two conditions since close observation will show them to be intimately intermingled in almost all cases. The chief seat of these spasms is the speech musculature, broadly envisioned, including the breathing apparatus, the larynx, and the muscles of the lips, tongue, and face, but the spasms are by no means limited to this field, as during blocked effort at speech it is often easy to see that many other muscular fields are in a greater or less degree of tonic spasm. The clonic spasms also may overflow into channels other than those actually needed for speech, giving rise to clonic movements of quite distant muscular groups. Occasionally also this motor overflow may result in short, jerky movements of the arm, foot, shoulder, or head which might very easily be interpreted as the movements of chorea or St. Vitus' dance. Differentiation from chorea is, however, simple since the movements here described are consistently associated with an effort at speech and often occur only while the child is actually blocked by a spasm, whereas true chorea shows no such association with the speech effort. These muscular responses in fields other than those employed in speech are, however, an exception, and commonly the more readily observable abnormal motor responses are limited to the face and particularly to the lips and tongue. Here a very wide variety of movements may be observed, for the most part represented as fragments. Thus at times during an effort at speech one may recognize movements of suckling, spitting, biting, laughing, crying, smiling, etc. Their range is very much wider than that of the suckling movements which have been so selectively stressed in some interpretations of their genesis.

When classified by the time of onset of the disorder, stuttering children fall into two main groups. Many show a speech impediment from the time they first begin to talk, that is, from two or three years of age; others develop a normal and facile speech which continues so until the sixth to eighth year, when stuttering begins. If we consider what is happening to the child's language development in these two critical periods we see that during the first—that is, at the age of two or three—he is just beginning to establish his habits of speech and also of handedness. Some delay in both the beginning of speech and in the preferential use of either hand is common in the history of children who begin to stutter at this age. The second critical period occurs when the child is just beginning to learn his graphic language—reading and writing—and beginning to integrate these new unilateral brain functions with his speech which is still in a somewhat formative stage.

It is very common to find a considerable measure of special writing disability coexisting with stuttering. Many childhood stutterers apparently have as much

Problems in Children

difficulty in acquiring writing as they had in speech. With that group of children whose stuttering started early, that is, with their first efforts at speech, a typical reading disability also frequently develops when they first enter school. This has occurred often enough in our series of cases so that we feel that special attention should be paid to the early reading training of a child who has been or is a stutterer.

When we classify the childhood stutterers on the basis of history and examinations of eyedness and handedness, we find that they fall into four main groups. The first is that in which an enforced shift from the left to the right hand has been carried out by parents or nurse. The second is comprised of those who have been slow in selecting a master hand and who on examination show marked motor intergrading. In the third there is no history of handedness shift and no evidence of intergrading on examination but a very strong family history of stuttering. The fourth group consists of cases in which there is no history of shift and no evidence of intergrading and which are said to be the only cases of stuttering in the family. In an occasional case no pertinent familial history can be obtained but in the majority of instances of these apparently sporadic cases, disorders of the language faculty of other types or the presence of a familial tendency toward left-handedness can be found by proper inquiry. Stuttering in children has no true counterpart in the syndromes caused by lesions occurring in the adult brain.

7. *Combined or Mixed Syndromes*

Emphasis has been given in the description of several of the foregoing developmental syndromes to the fact that they may be very highly selective and in this regard much more nearly approach the abstraction of a "pure" condition than do those which follow a lesion of the brain in the adult. In passing, mention has also been made of the occasional appearance of two developmental disorders in the same individual. Thus the child who stutters with his earliest speech is quite apt to encounter specific trouble with reading when he reaches that point in his schooling, and even more commonly will show a measure of the special writing disability. Inaccuracies in the auditory recall of word sounds comparable to a mild degree of word deafness have been identified as a complicating factor in many cases of the reading disability and even more strikingly in errors in spelling, as when a child mispronounces a word and then spells it as he has pronounced it. More serious combinations also occur, however. In those cases of severe word deafness which we have been able to follow into school, as well as in several which we have had under our own guidance in retraining, a strephosymbolic disturbance of comparatively severe grade has been revealed by their approach to reading and writing. When both of these conditions exist the problem of language training is doubly complex and the outlook for good intellectual progress is not particularly bright. Some of these children are skillful with their hands and do quite well in manual occupations. Some, however, exhibit a meas-

Problems in Children

ure of apraxia as well as word deafness and strephosymbolia, and here practically every channel of competition and advancement is blocked. At present it appears that any one of these major disorders may be strikingly improved by means of careful, detailed, individual diagnosis and appropriate instruction, but where all three pathways—the visual, the auditory, and the kinaesthetic—partake in a developmental delay or disorder, the task of training becomes almost too intricate for our present understanding and techniques.

HEREDITARY FACTORS

The occurrence of a case of developmental delay in acquiring language carries no inference as to the intellectual status of the family from which it sprang, nor would our observations indicate the presence of any consistent neurotic taint in these families. Among our patients are to be found the sons and daughters of successful doctors, lawyers, ministers, scientists, writers, linguists, college professors and businessmen. One factor to be found in these families which is of specific interest to us, however, is the frequent occurrence of two or more cases of language disability in the same family. This has long been noted in the past but always, we believe, with regard to the occurrence of the same syndrome in closely related individuals, that is, congenital word blindness in one family, stuttering in another, etc. Bearing in mind the hypothesis that these various language disorders may stem from a common origin and that this may be the result of intermixture of right- and left-sidedness tendencies, our case histories have for a number of years inquired not only into the whole range of language disorders discussed in this lecture but also into the presence of normal left-handers in the family, and when this is done the familial factors are much more impressive than when the history is limited to the occurrence of any one syndrome in the stock.

Certain of the disorders under discussion may follow true to type in a given family so that stuttering may occur in several subsequent generations, as may the reading disability, without the appearance of other frank disorders. In the great majority of such cases normal left-handers will be found in the same families, however. As with any recessive hereditary character, this may be difficult to trace, since few family records are complete enough to ascertain the facts beyond the living generations and even here the early facts of development of the older members of the family may have been forgotten and their natural bent may have been markedly altered by training. One interesting story comes to memory in this connection. This was a family in which a child had encountered a severe reading disability and in which no instance of left-handedness could be recalled. Somewhat later, however, the family visited the Scottish castle which was the ancestral home of the mother's forebears, and found everything there the reverse of the common building practice and clearly designed to meet the needs of a race of left-handed warriors, and the countryside was filled with tales of the left-handed McD's.

No dogmatic statement can be made concerning the method of inheritance of these disabilities since the in-

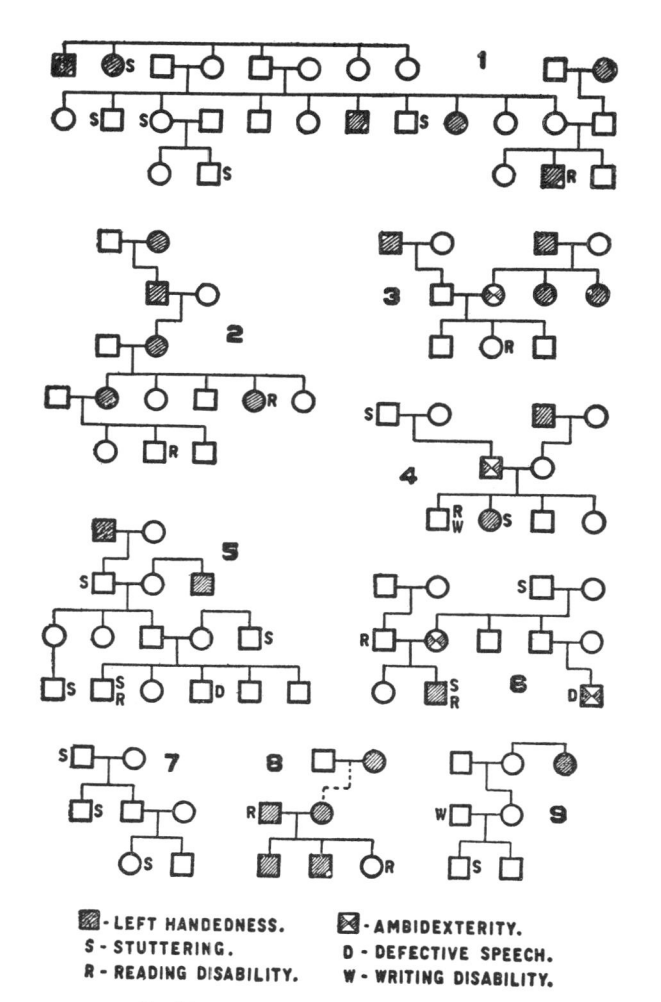

FIGURE 22. *Incidence of left-handedness and several types of language disorders in nine selected families.*

formation concerning the family backgrounds is too fragmentary for a careful analysis. However, it may be said that all of these difficulties in acquiring language are more frequent in boys than in girls. Our earlier work indicated that in strephosymbolia the ratio is about 3½ to 1 and the distribution among stutterers is probably approximately the same. This preponderance in males suggests a sex-influenced factor, although it is clearly not sex-linked. In our group of stutterers the transmission has been somewhat more frequent by the male parent while in strephosymbolia it seems somewhat more apt to follow the female line. These statements are tentative, however, and must await wider observation and analysis. The incidence of left-handedness and several varieties of language disorder in certain families is shown in Figure 22.

Since it has been necessary again to bring into our discussion the factor of left-handedness, it would seem wise to repeat the previous statement that there is no real reason to consider the straight left-handed individual in any way inferior to the right-handed except by reason of those inconveniences which are forced upon him by the custom and usage of the right-handed majority. It is only those in whom the tendency toward some measure of left-sidedness is present, but not in sufficient strength to assure complete unilateral superiority of the right hemisphere of the brain, in whom trouble may ensue and who form a fertile soil for the disturbing effects of misguided training.

EMOTIONAL REACTIONS AND BEHAVIOR PATTERNS

Since the children on whom our observations are here recorded were in the great majority of instances referred to us solely because of language delays or disorders, they form an unselected group as far as personality types and emotional and behavior problems are concerned, and we have seen a wide range of reaction patterns such as would be anticipated in any group so chosen. Because, however, of the cardinal importance of taking into consideration in any properly planned course of retraining, the emotional make-up of the child and his reaction to his particular disability, we have in history taking and in examination included as complete a study of the personality development of the child and the outstanding environmental factors in his situation as circumstances permitted. Especial attention has been given in each case to ascertaining whether there were any deviations in emotional development before the onset of the language difficulty and whether there has been any marked change in the child's behavior reactions at school or at home in the years that have followed. We have found, as would be expected, that there is a very considerable variability in the individual reaction to a given handicap dependent not only upon diverse factors in the child's own make-up but also upon the social, economic and educational status and ambitions of the family. It is obvious, for example, that a boy whose life ambition is to become an undertaker's helper and whose family approves this choice, as was the case with one of our patients, will not suffer from a reading disability so severely as will one who is bent on following his father into medicine, law, or teaching. Pressures arising within the family circle through competition with brothers and sisters may also influence his reactions. It is not uncommon to find a youngster who has shown no special concern over not being able to read in his second or third year in school until a younger brother or sister entering the first grade and finding reading easy, is able to surpass the older brother in a few months and then the trouble begins. The stress placed by the school on the child's disability also constitutes a definitive factor, and the general educational philosophy of the school as well as the achievement of the child's class as a whole and the personality of his individual teachers must be estimated in the evaluation of his emotional reactions.

As the child who carries any form of unrelieved language handicap grows older, there naturally ensues an accumulated emotional overlay which in many instances makes any effort to assign etiological significance to either the organic or the emotional factors that are then apparent in the situation as purposeless as attempting to allot pre-eminence to either the warp or the woof of a piece of cloth. From our experience with nearly a thousand cases of the various types of these developmental disorders it becomes clear that no generalization concerning the appearance of emotional disturbances in the various syndromes under discussion is possible. We may, however, briefly review the reactions which we have met most frequently in association with each disability when seen early in its course.

The *reading disability* cases as a group form a clear

cut example of the appearance of emotional disturbances which are purely secondary to the academic obstacle. The great majority of these children have exhibited no deviation in either their emotional or intellectual development up to the time they have encountered reading in their first or second year of school. Indeed, the usual story of parents and other observers is that of an entirely normal, healthy and happy child up to the age of six or seven, who entered upon his school life with eager anticipation and had no difficulty in adjustments throughout the nursery school or kindergarten periods. The primary teachers may, moreover, have made no attempt to force him to read, but no matter how carefully the school attempts to capitalize those things in which the child is successful and minimize his failures, he cannot be shielded from making a comparison of his own between the rate at which he is learning to read and that of his classmates, and he tends to develop an entirely natural feeling of inferiority as a result. At first this may be limited strictly to the subjects of reading and spelling and if proper treatment for these delays is instituted early it will not extend beyond this boundary and will also be rapidly eradicated there with progress in the remedial work. When, however, proper treatment is not instituted or the handicap is entirely disregarded because of the "laissez faire" attitude adopted by many schools, the feeling of inferiority is very apt to extend to other fields so that the child approaches every task with the expectation of failure, and all of his school work may lag seriously behind. At times indeed this may tincture his whole reaction pattern. One of my third grade pupils who could read nothing and whose younger brother in first grade was learning to read easily, when asked to help his father with some simple tasks around the house, replied, "Oh, I can't do that, Dad, you know I'm a dumb-bell." In others a generalized feeling of depression has developed with unwonted tearfulness both at home and at school or an attitude of extreme dejection.

We have studied a number of children in whom the failure has led to a striking emotional blocking of expression. This also is at first apt to be restricted to reading and spelling and the child will talk freely and easily about his arithmetic or the facts that he has learned in his geography class but will stop abruptly the moment reading becomes the topic. At times this blocking extends to all his work at school and may even include the athletic program there, so that the boy cannot be led into any discussion of school or its activities. Not infrequently the child shows on the surface a cultivated indifference which masks the depth of feeling which exists toward his reading trouble until this is revealed by the marked relief of emotional tension which follows the beginning of successful treatment. Occasionally the strephosymbolics show a definite frustration reaction when their repeated attempts at reading have been unsuccessful, although they seem somewhat more apt to attempt to cover up their shortcomings and evade as many reading demands as they can. We have seen others who have reacted to their difficulty by the adoption of a boisterous, swaggering attitude, assuring us that reading was their favorite and best subject in spite of the fact that they were failing completely in it. Emotional instability resulting in the so-called "nervous" or "high-strung" reaction pattern

Problems in Children

in which distractibility and difficulty in concentration are outstanding has been observed in some of the reading disability cases, but except in the few in whom this was traceable back to infancy, this tendency has promptly disappeared with the institution of a successful program of teaching. We have not observed any tendency toward seclusiveness and phantasia or the presence of abnormal fears or undue dependence on maternal protection as characteristic of the strephosymbolics. Indeed, time and again, the parents report that the child with the reading disability is the best adjusted and the most dependable member of the entire family group.

With the cases of reading disability encountered somewhat later in their school progress, the feeling of inferiority is apt to be marked as a result of their repeated failures, although this may to some extent be offset in those who have a good innate intelligence and are able to compete successfully with their fellows in mathematics and science. Compensations of this and other types, such as good athletic skills and social acceptability, naturally play a large part in determining the severity of the inferiority reaction in a given child. When an adequate program of retraining has been instituted and is proving to the child that he can make progress against his mysterious handicap, the inferiority feelings usually gradually evaporate. While carefully guided retraining has been successful in a technical sense in teaching reading to those who have even severe degrees of strephosymbolia, one might almost say that the greatest profit from such a program comes not so much in the reading advance, which at best must be slow, as in the effect which this improvement brings about in the child's personality. Relief from emotional tension, a generally more buoyant frame of mind and regained self-confidence are by-products of no mean value.

The cases of selective *writing disability* show no striking emotional accompaniment. These children are usually somewhat ashamed of their lack of writing skill and often no little puzzled by it, particularly when they are deft in drawing or in using tools, but as a rule this defect is not so consistently exposed to others as is a difficulty with speech or even one in reading, and ordinarily there is engendered in the child no striking emotional deviation. Nor do they as a group show any personality characteristics which mark them off from any chance group of children except in the cases of those in whom the writing disability exists as a complication of others of these difficulties such as an inability to read, a speech defect, or an apraxia. If very severe in degree, however, it may lead to failures in written examinations which the child may consider unjust, and he may develop a resentment toward his teachers or a feeling of frustration.

Since the beginning of the handicap assessed against the child in *developmental word deafness* reaches so far back into infancy, it is difficult to determine what characteristics are innate in this group and what are developed as a result of the defect. We will therefore merely describe the emotional patterns which we have observed without attempt at assigning them value. As a group these children are very slow in gaining a normal measure of independence of their parents, and several whom we have seen have been quite fearful of any strange person or situation. Negativism beyond

Problems in Children

that which might be due to failure to comprehend spoken commands has not been found with any consistency in these cases. Temper tantrums of an explosive sort have been observed as a part of the behavior pattern in several word deaf children. It would seem as though the earlier infantile pattern of screaming to gain a desire has persisted here through lack of the normal substitution of the growing ability to express desires in words. One boy of eight who had a marked deficit in word understanding launched a vigorous and somewhat successful physical attack on the headmaster of his school when criticized for the infraction of minor rules. Extensive experience in retraining this boy over a considerable period of time uncovered no tendency toward recurrence of this type of outburst when care was taken to make sure that the boy understood just what was asked of him and why, and our ultimate interpretation of his assault on the headmaster was that of a belligerent panic in the face of a verbal criticism which he could not readily understand. The notably bellicose attitude toward his fellow pupils contained in the history of one of our cases of severe high frequency deafness with considerable interference with word perception again seemed to link this pugnacious behavior with difficulty in understanding spoken words.

In cases of word deafness, maternal overprotection as judged by standards for other children is usual and would seem to be a natural consequence of the longer period of dependence on others through which these children must pass before gaining sufficient mastery of words for understanding or for self-expression. Naturally, a mother who realizes that her child is not developing as he should and cannot make his wants known to others will continue to anticipate his needs, and this in turn minimizes the child's necessity for speech and in such a situation it not infrequently becomes necessary to place the general training of the child in entirely new hands before specific measures aimed at his disability can be profitably undertaken.

In sharp contrast to the cases of special reading disability, these children with an obstacle to the understanding of the spoken word do not seem to show any marked feeling of inferiority. Unless a considerable measure of spontaneous improvement occurs or unless training methods prove efficacious, they suffer from a progressive deficit in the concepts and ideas which are ordinarily absorbed without effort through conversation with others, but they seem to lack insight into this defect very much as the generally defective children do. There does not seem to be, however, in those whom we have studied, any retardation in emotional maturation or any serious fault in judgment such as accompanies feeblemindedness. Within the limits of their understanding they give the impression of being rather competent individuals.

Since the word deaf child cannot understand the speech of others and cannot express himself he is rather apt to play alone when young, but this does not seem to be an inherent seclusiveness and some of this group have shown definite social inclinations and a tendency toward garrulousness within their limitation.

The cases of *motor speech delay* which we have studied have shown a quiet, friendly shyness. They are quite ready to respond to advances from others and do not actively withdraw from social contacts,

Problems in Children

but their difficulty in expressing themselves naturally prevents them from taking the initiative toward making new friends among children or adults. As a group they have shown no abnormal fears nor signs of marked seclusiveness, although their difficulty in making themselves understood often leads to marked frustration reactions and occasionally to related explosive behavior. There is naturally a tendency for their mothers to look after them closely because of their inability to talk and sometimes a reluctance to undertake any disciplinary training since a two-way discussion of situations is impossible, but on the whole they do not appear to be inclined to be overdependent or very different, emotionally, from other children of their age.

The children with *developmental apraxia* are cautious in undertaking new motor activities, but in view of their disability this appears more in the light of a good understanding of their own capacities than as an abnormally fearful disposition. They all show as they grow older a marked feeling of inferiority but it must be borne in mind that in all athletic activities they *are* inferior so that such feelings are closely akin to insight. Some of them are very persevering in their attempts to overcome their handicap and reasonably successful in doing so. The apraxics occasionally are apt at scholastic work and gain a variable degree of compensation from this. They are often socially acceptable to the group in spite of their gawkiness and apparently are not inherently seclusive.

The picture in *children who stutter* shows a striking contrast to that in adults with this impediment, as has been stated previously in this volume.

In the younger group—those who begin to stutter

with their first efforts at speech—there is no consistently unusual trend in emotional development. They are not as a rule overdependent on their parents or antagonistic to them; they develop the usual interest in social contacts with other children of their own age and are not emotionally unstable except for an occasional explosive outburst as a result of the frustration of their efforts at speech. These explosions, however, are impersonal and not aimed at parents, teachers, or companions and give the impression of a form of protest to their disability. In contrast to the emotionally equable temperament of the majority of these children they show a rather marked degree of hyperkinesis or motor tension. Their movements are apt to be abrupt and sometimes jerky in character so that they are frequently described as "nervous" children. Some of these movements are directly associated with the speech effort and are to be considered as associated movements or motor overflows which have already been discussed, but there is in addition a tendency for the stuttering child to display a considerable degree of general motor activity. It would seem important to differentiate this form of "nervousness" from the emotional lability which also goes under the same rather vague term.

In the older group—those whose speech difficulty first develops from six to eight years of age—there is usually a history of entirely normal development—physical, emotional, and intellectual—up to this critical age, and commonly there is no history of adequate trauma either physical or psychological to account for the onset of the stuttering. Usually during the first year or more of their speech disorder they show none of

Problems in Children

the personality scars which characterize the adult with this affliction. As a group they are not unusually fearful —indeed some are adventurous—nor is there at first any evidence of the fear of speaking which may be so prominent later. They often on the contrary are naturally talkative and very persistent in their efforts at speech and in no wise inhibited from making an attempt to talk, although some of those whose disorder is characterized by long blocks in which no sound is forthcoming seem to be more prone to submit resignedly to the difficulty in talking and to curtail markedly their speech output. Clearly the problem in these childhood stutterers is far different from that of adults who stutter, and calls not only for specific treatment of the disorder itself but for measures aimed at the prevention of the various personality disorders and emotional maladjustment which bulk so large in the picture of this condition when seen in the adult.

Chapter Three

INTERPRETATION AND TREATMENT OF CERTAIN DISORDERS OF LANGUAGE IN CHILDREN

IN the first chapter of this volume certain of the disturbances of language which follow injury to the brain in the adult were briefly reviewed and attention was called to the arresting fact that these disorders may follow a lesion in one hemisphere of the brain but only if it be the master half of the brain which is injured. It was further pointed out that our only guide to the master hemisphere in the adult was his laterality, and observations in children were reported which indicate a wide range of variability in establishing a clear cut laterality as measured by tests and history of development of handedness, eyedness, and footedness.

In the second chapter five syndromes of delay or disorder in the acquisition of language were described—developmental alexia, special disability in writing, developmental word deafness, motor speech delay, and stuttering—and one other—developmental apraxia—which follows the same unilateral pattern of organization in the brain although it does not always interfere with language development. In all but one of these six disorders, viz., stuttering, it was pointed out that the symptoms observed are a very exact counterpart of those seen in the corresponding syndromes in the adult,

Problems in Children 143

suggesting strongly that the determiner for these disabilities in childhood is very closely related physiologically to that which is disturbed by lesions in the critical cortices controlling language in the adult. Since the normal pattern in the adult is a concentration of control of the functions under discussion in the hemisphere opposite to the master hand, and since our clinical observations show so wide a variation both in time and degree in the development of a selective preference for either side in many children, it is suggested that these disorders in language development may derive from a comparable variation affecting the essential language areas of the brain and thus rest on a basis largely physiological in nature and not dependent on defect or destruction of any part of the cortex.

The present chapter offers a discussion of the neurological interpretation of the children's disorders, a general review of the principles on which our experiments in retraining have been founded, and a brief discussion of the specific methods of treatment employed in each syndrome. A word of caution must be entered here, and that is that no general formula can be given which will be applicable to all cases of any of the syndromes discussed. Each case of developmental delay forms an individual problem in which factors derived from the neurological status, the emotional reactions, the educational needs and the facilities for carrying on retraining must be evaluated and a program devised to conform to all of these. This point can scarcely be emphasized enough since we are all prone to search for a simplified and universally applicable formula, but no such general "method" can be defined for any of these syndromes and any attempt to apply such a blanket prescription without thorough diagnosis of the individual case would assuredly lead to error and misguided effort.

INTERPRETATION

As has already been mentioned, these special disabilities occurring in children may show a much higher selectivity than do the corresponding syndromes in the adult. In certain of them, notably the reading disability, we are able to observe the step by step evolution of the disorder from the simplest beginnings, and moreover it is thrown into bold relief against the entirely normal previous progress of the child in his general intellectual and emotional development and against normal or even superior accomplishment in spoken language. Thus the problems presented are much less complex than those encountered in the tangled wreckage of a group of closely interrelated functions such as we see in the acquired aphasias. Apparently in the normal literate adult there is an intimate interweaving between such fractions of the language faculty as reading, writing, spelling, and speaking, which results in more or less functional overlapping, so that the results of even the most restricted brain damage are apt to be complex and rarely if ever do we see pure syndromes such as can be demonstrated in some of the developmental disorders in children. For this reason this group offer a particularly favorable field for investigation of the language function.

From our studies, extending over the past ten years, of the symptoms of the six disorders under discussion we have so far been able to recognize only one factor

Problems in Children

which is common to the entire group and that is a difficulty in repicturing or rebuilding in the order of presentation, sequences of letters, of sounds, or of units of movement and a brief presentation of our observations of this factor in the various syndromes is presented here because it has served to guide many of our experiments in treatment.

The reading disability cases are sufficiently advanced intellectually when they encounter their trouble so that they can be very intensively studied and it is clear that this disorder is not one of sensory reception but rather of memory. By a variety of tests it is possible to show that these children see the word that they are attempting to read correctly, but that the record left by previous exposures to the same word is not sufficiently clear to suffice for its recognition, as in reading, and still less so for its reproduction, as in spelling. The most apt demonstration of this point is that a child will frequently misread a word which he has just copied correctly and will still more often misspell such a word. When we study the errors made by these children in attempting to read and even more strikingly when we analyze their efforts at spelling, we see that the major interference with the process of recognizing or recalling the word is a failure to repicture the exact order of its constituent letters. As these children are progressively exposed to reading and spelling instruction, especially in the milder cases, this disorderly recall of sequences becomes somewhat less clear cut since they gradually learn to recognize many words correctly, particularly when clues to their meaning are offered in the context. In those children whose training in reading has been exclusively by the "whole word" or "sight method," however, order remains as an obvious difficulty much longer than in those who have been taught the sounds which each letter represents and hence have an auditory clue to the proper sequence. The characteristic confusions by reason of reversed orientation and reversed sequence which lead to the misreading of *b* for *d* and *was* for *saw* form a special instance which will be elaborated later in this chapter.

In the cases of special writing disability in children, as outlined in the previous chapter, there is sometimes difficulty in forming the individual letters but the purer cases are frequently able to form each character exactly and with ease but find an immediate difficulty when they attempt to combine them into sequences, whether connected as in cursive writing or separated as in "manuscript" writing, and thus, except in those children with an apraxic factor who have a very low degree of skill in finger movements and those whose native skill has been sacrificed through enforced training of the wrong hand, the chief obstacle in cases of the special writing disability is in the formation of sequences of letters by which the word is constructed.

Naturally, since the syndromes of developmental word blindness and developmental word deafness are so closely comparable in every respect, we were led to look for reversals in the order of the speech sounds in cases of the latter condition and a few such distortions have been observed as when a child used the word *naf* for *fan,* for example. Reversed order of parts of the sounds in a word as in *emeny* for *enemy* and *pomerad* for *promenade* is somewhat more common as is the transposition of the two parts of paired or

Problems in Children

associated words as when "cuff buttons" is recalled as "button cuffs" or when a boy reports that he lives on "Driverside River." This form of error has not been common in our studies however and by far the more frequent type is due to irregular distortions in order of reproduction of the component sound units of a word, often combined with the omission of some of its sounds. Usually the first few sounds are given correctly while those toward the end are distorted in order or slurred or omitted. Occasionally these alterations give rise to neologisms such as those that have already been quoted from the speech of an eighteen-year-old, word deaf boy. While these children show many errors of a wide variety of kinds it is clear that their difficulty is not in hearing and not in the speech mechanism but in the recalling of words previously heard, for the purpose of recognizing them when heard again or for use in speech, and that one of the outstanding obstacles to such recall is remembering all of the sounds in a word and these sounds in their proper order. This can be demonstrated in some cases of developmental word deafness by the fact that the child is able to echo correctly many words which he cannot recall in expression, and indeed a prolonged period of echolalia is common in this disorder. During this period the child automatically repeats many of the words and even phrases and sentences which are spoken to him but which he cannot produce except as an echo. As will be seen, this forms an interesting parallel to the ability of the word blind cases to copy words which they can neither read nor spell.

In the case of vision, which is the function of paramount importance in reading, the correct revival requires proper spatial orientation and spatial sequences —that is, the symbols constituting the printed word must be recalled in the proper order in space—while in audition, on the other hand, we are concerned entirely with a temporal factor—that is, the sounds must follow each other in the correct order in time—and it is the recall of sounds in proper temporal sequence which seems to be at fault in word deafness.

In those children who are delayed in learning to talk but who seem to have a normal understanding of the speech of others, we again meet with a difficulty in sequence building which is as striking as that in any of the syndromes so far discussed from this viewpoint. Mention has already been made, in the description of the syndrome of motor speech delay, of the ability of children with this disorder to echo many sounds which they cannot use in speech. Indeed, many of them can reproduce as an echo all of the sounds of the letters of the alphabet but cannot make use of these same sounds in words and may not be able even to echo short blended series of sounds, and it is this sequential blending which seems to constitute the greater part of their difficulty in acquiring propositional speech.

In the case of children who have great trouble in learning complex patterns of movement—the developmental apraxias—simpler movements are often readily acquired although they may be lacking in grace or smoothness. Here the controlling sensory element is that of kinaesthesis or the registration of movement patterns. In by far the great majority of body movements, while one side is carrying out one stage of the act, the other is co-operating or preparing itself for

Problems in Children 149

the next stage or phase and a closely co-ordinated control of the two sides is essential. In many of the simpler acts, such as walking, there is evidence to suggest that much of this co-ordination is carried out by the spinal cord and other nervous structures below the level of the brain. When, however, we attempt to interrupt the simple movement pattern of walking and use parts of it to reassemble into a dance step, for example, this new combination is without question controlled by the brain and it is in just such recombinations of simple movement units into new sequential patterns that the apraxic child encounters trouble.

In stuttering children we frequently find true phonetic disorders in that certain letter sounds are imperfectly made or cannot be produced at all, but this is not always true and some of these children have as good a grasp of the process of forming the individual sounds as have normal speakers of the same age. Stuttering is so exceedingly variable in its severity from time to time in the same patient and so strikingly different in its expression in different patients that any general statement is hazardous and may readily be met with exceptions. We may risk this hazard, however, by pointing out that at least a major part of the young stutterer's trouble lies not in saying any one sound but in moving on to the next. Thus while we usually say that the individual is stuttering on the *k* sound in K-K-Katy, he is in reality saying *k* correctly over and over again and his difficulty actually lies in changing from the motor pattern needed for *k* to that necessary for the next sound, *a*. Thus in this disturbance of speech also, the fusing of the simple sound units into word-blends seems to play a prominent, if not the commanding, role.

While this difficulty with the revival of sequences affecting recognition in the two sensory syndromes—reading and the understanding of speech—and affecting reproduction in the motor syndromes—motor speech delay, agraphia, stuttering, and apraxia—is the only factor which we have been able to find common to the symptomatology of the group as a whole, and while it throws little or no light on the genesis of these disorders, yet there are several facts to be observed in the strephosymbolics and the developmental agraphics which challenge us to a neurological explanation. I refer here to the characteristic tendency to reversals in reading and spelling found in the strephosymbolics; to the development, without training, of a facility in mirror reading in the same group, and to the occasional occurrence, again without training, of a skill in mirror writing in cases with a selective writing disability.

The reversals are of two types. First, those in which confusion exists between two letters with the same form but opposite orientation, as when *b* is confused with *d*, and *p* with *q*. These we have called static reversals. The second is when there is an element of sinistrad progression through a series of letters as when *was* is read as *saw*, or *tomorrow* as *tworrom*. These we have called kinetic reversals. The two types are practically always to be found associated in any case of strephosymbolia, but they vary markedly both in their relative frequence and in the resistance which they offer to eradication by retraining. That the reversals play a significant role in strephosymbolia is adequately sup-

Problems in Children

ported by our earlier studies in Iowa. The errors made by a group of reading disability cases were tabulated and compared with those made by a carefully selected control group of normal readers of the same reading grade and intelligence, and the errors by reversal were found to be significant statistically for the reading disability cases at each of the first four reading grades which were studied. Not only was this so, but the frequence with which errors by reversal appeared in the work of a given case proved to correlate with the amount of his retardation in reading, that is, with the severity of his disorder. In mirror reading likewise, the relative success achieved by the strephosymbolics was significant when compared with a carefully selected control group and it was noted that as the child progressed in dextrad reading, his skill in mirror reading was comparably reduced.

One fact about the reversals which will bear emphasis is the apparent equivalence to the child of the dextrad and sinistrad patterns. Thus there is no consistency in the errors made here and either one of the twin letters may be at one moment called by its right name and at the next by that of its opposite. Again, we must take cognizance of the fact that both mirror reading and mirror writing skills may exist in selected cases as a by-product of their attempts to learn to read or write in the dextrad direction and without specific training in the sinistrad forms. It is evident in the untrained mirror reading skill shown by some strephosymbolics that during attempts to learn to read words in the dextrad direction the brain has registered these words in the sinistrad position as well, so that they have become serviceable for recognition of the mirrored copy, and similarly in certain cases of the special writing disability, while efforts at teaching the dextrad or ordinary direction of writing have met with little or no success, the brain has received and registered the mirrored forms with such fidelity that mirror writing of a very acceptable quality has been possible with no instruction and no practice.

Since in the normal adult the cortices governing the language functions are active in only one hemisphere of the brain, it is pertinent to inquire concerning the physiological conditions existing in corresponding areas of the other half. Here we have very little exact information. The gyri of the non-dominant hemisphere corresponding to those which form the critical areas for the control of language are a part of what are known to neurologists as "the silent areas" since injury to them gives rise to no outstanding symptoms. They are however almost, if not quite, as well developed in size and in nerve cell and fiber connections as are those of the dominant half, and we must assume therefore that they receive and register nerve impulses with practically the same freedom as do those of the controlling hemisphere. The fact that the normal functional pattern in control of reading is a strictly unilateral one, as demonstrated by acquired alexia, infers therefore that any registrations which may have occurred in the non-dominant hemisphere have been elided or are unused. In recent years there has been a tendency to question the existence of exact sensory records in the brain and to speak in vague terms of dynamic forces here, and the term engram, which means a physiological record, is said to have "gone out of fashion," particularly in the psychological literature. However it is

Problems in Children 153

self-evident that any form of learning presupposes the storage in the brain of some sort of a record of a stimulus which will permit recognition when the same stimulus is encountered again, and the writer prefers to retain the word engram to define such a record, and the facts which have been recorded here suggest very strongly that engrams exist in the non-dominant hemisphere which may, if not completely elided, cause confusion in recognition and recall. This view implies that the records established in the right and left brain hemispheres are oppositely oriented.

Strictly opposite right and left orientation cannot be questioned in the motor structures. That the bones, muscles, joints and nerves of the left arm and hand, for example, are the mirrored opposites of those of the right is categorical, and this strict antitropism or right and left pairing can also be readily demonstrated in the nerve cell mechanisms which control the movements of the limbs. Thus a microscopic examination of the spinal cord at the level at which the motor nerves to the arms arise will show groups of the large nerve cells which are directly in command of muscular movements arranged on either side of the midline in the same number and in the same patterns but in mirrored design. (Figure 23) This same plan is carried out in that part of the brain cortex which in its turn directs the activity of the motor cells in the spinal cord in voluntary motion. Here the giant nerve cells of Betz are arranged in similar order in the two hemispheres but again as strict right- and left-hand opposites. Immediately behind the motor cortex of the brain lies the field in which messages from the skin bringing information as to the place of origin on the body surface of stimuli of pain, touch and temperature are recorded, and in this same general field the kinaesthetic stimuli from muscles, joints and tendons are also received. That the registration of these groups of incoming messages must also be in the nature of right and left ori-

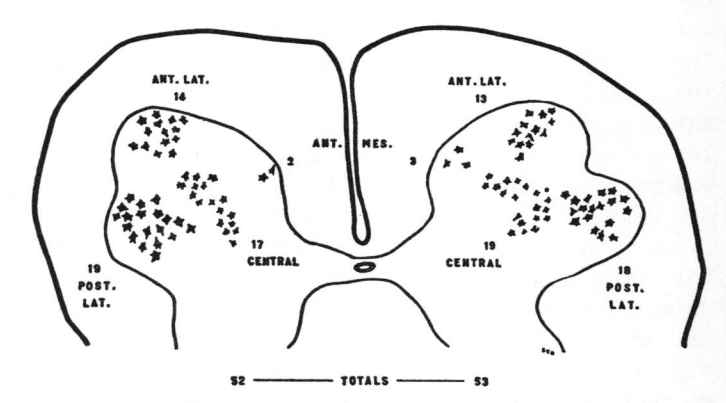

FIGURE 23. *Projection drawing of a cross-section of the spinal cord to show the strict antitropic arrangement of the motor nerve cells of the right and left halves of the cord.*

ented engrams is entirely obvious since they must coordinate with the similarly oriented motor mechanisms to give adequate control. Other considerations bear out this statement that the kinaesthetic and common sensory records in the brain are oppositely oriented.

In the field of vision the situation is not so clear, but as far as the gross brain structure in the areas which subserve this function is concerned, there is just as strict right and left pairing as is to be found in the motor and kinaesthetic areas. In other words, the brain contains right and left visual areas which are exactly alike except for their opposite orientation and we feel therefore that the question of the existence in the non-dominant hemisphere of engrams of opposite orientation from those in the dominant hemisphere cannot be lightly dismissed as the probable source of the static and kinetic reversals and of the spontaneous ability in mirror reading and mirror writing.

Since the problem of heredity plays such an important part in the genesis of the special language disabilities as well as in the problem of right- and left-handedness it may be well to discuss briefly the ways in which it might operate. We cannot at present accept the hereditary transmission of a purely functional character and believe that the passing on from the family stock of a strong preference for the use of the right or the left hand must rest on the transmission of a better brain structure in the left or right hemisphere, respectively, which in turn leads to the development of a functional superiority. As yet we have no precise knowledge on this point. Many investigators hold that in the adult the hemisphere of the brain opposite to the master hand, which is also the dominant hemisphere for language in almost all cases, is somewhat larger than that of the non-dominant. So far as the writer's own studies have gone they do not support this view and we have no accurate information concerning the relative size of the two hemispheres at birth or in infancy. Moreover, size in the brain is a treacherous guide as may be readily seen by consideration of the recorded brain weights of various men of genius. This is true largely because a very considerable part of the brain's bulk is composed of materials which are not primarily concerned in its functional integrity—notably the fatty insulating sheaths which surround nerve fibers. Functional aptitude is probably dependent more on numbers of nerve cells, richness of their interconnections and abundance of blood supply than on the total size of the nervous organs, and it is therefore quite possible that either the left or right brain hemisphere might be endowed by heredity with a physical superiority over its mate without differing from it appreciably in size. Regardless, however, of the ultimate answer to this question, it is apparent that such structural superiority as is passed on to a given child might encompass the entire hemisphere or might be found in one area only and through usage lead to the development of a functional superiority of the whole hemisphere on that side, or as a third possibility the child might be endowed with a better structure in the cortex of one brain area in one brain hemisphere and in other areas on the opposite side, leading to a difficulty in establishing a complete unilateral superiority in functional use. Some considerations of the clinical observations made in cases of the special disabilities would suggest that the third condition may obtain, but no solution to these problems can be expected until much wider neuroanatomical, neurophysiological and neuropathological studies have been carried out.

TREATMENT

Experiments in treatment were incorporated as an integral part of our first program of research into these developmental delays and disorders of the acquisition of language with the hope that such investiga-

Problems in Children

tion might throw more light upon the basic problems of their genesis which have already been discussed in this volume as well as with the more practical aim of finding means of aiding these children to overcome their handicaps. These experiments which at first were restricted largely to cases of the reading disability and stuttering were initiated in 1927 in the Iowa State Psychopathic Hospital under a grant from the Rockefeller Foundation. The writer there began the extension of this investigation to the other syndromes and this wider experimental program was carried forward as the Language Research Project of the New York Neurological Institute between 1930 and 1936. Because of the novelty of the clinical material, many cases encountered in private practice have also served as research material both from the standpoint of improved diagnosis and as a means of evaluating methods of retraining. From these varied sources we have now had the opportunity of studying carefully almost a thousand cases representing all ages from the preschool child to the college student and including pupils from public, private and parochial schools and from schools representing every shade of educational philosophy from the most progressive to the ultra-conservative.

As has already been stated, each child presents an individual problem, not only because of the diverse influence of a considerable number of environmental conditions, but also because the relative part played by each of the three major functions entering into the language faculty—vision, audition, and kinaesthesis—varies markedly in different children as does the child's emotional reaction to his difficulty. The first step toward successful treatment therefore must be a careful evaluation of the extrinsic factors—economic, social, educational, etc.—together with an extensive analysis of the status of spoken language, graphic language, motor skills or limitations, and emotional reactions. Our experiences in teaching reading to those children who have suffered from a delay or defect in learning this subject have pointed to the importance of sequence building in such cases and in our experiments in the other syndromes this has led us to look for such units as the child can use without difficulty in the field of his particular disability and to direct our training toward developing the process of fusing these smaller, available units into larger and more complex wholes. A brief review will be given here of the way in which this principle has been applied to each syndrome.

1. Developmental Alexia

The hallmark of the specific reading disability or strephosymbolia is a failure in recognition of a printed word even after it has been encountered many times. Because of this and because the great majority of the children whom we studied had already been unsuccessfully exposed to the sight or flash-card method of teaching reading, we believed it unnecessary to experiment extensively with this procedure and indeed as our observations were extended we came to feel not only that repeated flash exposure of the whole word was not effective but that it might in certain children even increase the tendency to confusion and failures of recognition. Since the majority of the cases of reading disability have shown a normal development of spoken

Problems in Children

language and could readily understand, when spoken to them, the same words which they could not read, our approach has been an attempt to capitalize their auditory competence by teaching them the phonetic equivalents of the printed letters and the process of blending sequences of such equivalents so that they might produce for themselves the spoken form of the word from its graphic counterpart. Since, moreover, in the greater number of strephosymbolics there is no frank disorder in the kinaesthetic function, we have made use of movement patterns to aid in eradicating confusions between twin letters and in maintaining consistent dextrad progress in assembling the units of the word. Thus in those children with moderate degrees of confusion who are seen during the first or second year of school and even at a much later period in cases of extreme severity, to eliminate the "static reversals" which lead to great insecurity in differentiating b's and d's and p's and q's and occasionally other somewhat less exactly antitropic letter forms such as f and t and a and s, the kinaesthetic pattern for each letter is established by having the child trace it over a pattern drawn by the teacher, at the same time giving its sound or phonetic equivalent so that the sound of a letter b, for example, is being produced simultaneously with the movement required to draw this symbol. The obvious purpose of this procedure is to fix the association of the sound with the properly oriented letter form, and its efficacy usually becomes apparent shortly after such exercises have been begun by the fact that the child can, by using the motion, consistently differentiate the confused pairs long before he can be sure of them by visual inspection alone. Our first attention is given to fixing the mnemonic linkage between "what the letter says," i.e., its *sound,* and the properly oriented printed form, but since the letter *name* must also be available to the child for use in oral spelling, this is also taught in the same way. Ordinarily the tracing while sounding is not indicated for teaching the sounds of the letters other than those mentioned above, although occasionally other letter confusions such as *h* and *k* and *u* and *n* are profitably eradicated by the same procedure. It has proved impossible to forecast the amount of practice in tracing-sounding which will be required for a given child. In general, the tendency to confusion in orientation varies with the severity of the disability but it is also strikingly inconstant in the same child from day to day. Even after the task of telling the twin letters apart seems to have been mastered, a reversion to the former uncertainty frequently occurs. At times this can be related to fatigue, to an oncoming cold or to some unusual emotional stress, but at other times no clear cut reason can be discerned for the relapse. Since such a resurgence of the difficulty is common, however, we have found it advisable to check occasionally on the security with which these letters can be recognized and associated with their proper sounds and to repeat the tracing-sounding when any hesitation or uncertainty reappears. The emotional reaction of the child to this process as well as the success of the teacher in interesting the pupil in the end result of the practice are apparently factors of major importance in its rapid success.

No attempt will be made here to give details of the exact drill procedures which have been employed in establishing the phonetic basis for reading. We have

Problems in Children

tried to avoid overstandardization lest the procedure become too inflexible and be looked upon as a routine method applicable to all cases of non-readers, which would be clearly unwise in view of the wide variation in symptomatology and hence in training needs which these children exhibit. In teaching the phonetic units we have often found it convenient to use cards, each bearing a single letter or one of the more common digraphs, phonograms or diphthongs, printed by hand with fairly large rubber type in the lower case or small letter form. These cards are exposed to the child one at a time with instruction in "what it says" as well as its name, until he can give either the sound or name for any of the cards at sight. A question which often arises here is that of how far differentiation of the varying sounds of one vowel should be taught, and since our aim is merely to approximate the sounds closely enough so that a word known by ear will be recognized when read, we have found the finer distinctions quite unnecessary and have thus been able to keep the number of sounds to be learned from undue expansion.

One point of difficulty which we have encountered many times with the phonetic approach as it is usually taught is the tendency to stress the vowel component of a consonant sound so that the child produces $b\breve{u}$ for the sound of b with the major accent on the $\breve{u}$. This frequently makes trouble at the next step of the process when the blending of sounds is begun, since "bat" for such a child becomes "bŭ-ă-tŭ." Purification of the sounds of many of the consonants to avoid the $\breve{u}$ component is often difficult unless the child be taught from the beginning that b, for example, is $b\breve{u}$ only when followed by *ŭ*. Practice in combining the consonants with all of the child's available vowel sounds thus becomes the first step in the process of fusing or blending sound units into words.

It cannot be too strongly emphasized that simply teaching the child to be able to give the sounds for each letter of the alphabet and for the phonograms, etc., is hopelessly inadequate for his needs. We have repeatedly seen children referred to us as reading disability cases with the statement that the phonetic method had been tried but had failed. In these cases examination has revealed the fact that while the teaching of the phonetic equivalents may have been fairly complete, the next and most cardinal step, that of teaching the blending of the letter sounds in the exact sequence in which they occur in the word, had not been attempted or had been poorly carried out. It is this process of synthesizing the word as a spoken unit from its component sounds that often makes much more difficulty for the strephosymbolic child than do the static reversals and letter confusions. Here appear in the early cases and those of extreme severity the confusion in direction of sequences which has been presented as one of the diagnostic signs of strephosymbolia under the head of "kinetic reversals." It has already been mentioned that the two types of reversals do not always appear in the same numerical relation—in some children the *b-d* and *p-q* confusions have been found to be much more frequent than the definite progress to the left in attempting to read a word. However, in all of our very severe cases the tendency to sinistrad reading of parts or all of many words has been striking enough to demand special attention in the retrain-

Problems in Children

ing program, and this is even more apparent if we add those instances in which distorted order, other than frank reversals, is found in attempts to assemble the sounds of a word. We have found nonsense material particularly helpful with those children who have already learned to recognize many short words at sight but who are insecure at this and apt to misread words by the substitution of another with a somewhat similar general configuration. Nonsense syllables can be constructed of three or four letters and later these may be further combined into longer aggregates and the child is informed that they are not real words and that he must solve them by sounding without attempting to produce anything with which he is familiar.

With those children who are seen in the first year of their schooling and who hence are beginning to blend only very short series of sounds to correspond with very simple sequences of printed symbols we have found that the habit of consistent dextrad progress may develop with the sounding-out process and not require adjuvant procedures, although even in these cases the addition of a single letter to syllables of familiar length or the addition of one or more syllables to the sequence may lead to the appearance of the reversal tendency. Thus a child who has mastered direction in three letter words may have trouble with those containing four or may maintain the proper direction in the first syllable of a dissyllabic word and distort the second part or may follow in the proper direction through each of two syllables but assemble the syllables themselves in reversed order. In attempting to establish the habit of constant progress toward the right in these children, we have again experimented with the employment of movement as a guide and have had them point to the letters of the word with the finger as they progressed with the assembly of its sounds. This method of finger pointing while reading is a spontaneous act with some children and has been criticized as retarding the rate of reading seriously. There remains, however, the very pertinent question as to whether children who use finger pointing while reading are slow readers because of this habit or whether they are slow readers because of strephosymbolic confusions and make use of the finger to overcome their difficulty. It must be remembered here, moreover, that in the case of extreme degrees of the reading disability our choice may not lie between rapid and slow reading but between slow reading or none at all.

In the case of facile readers the acquisition and exercise of this skill brings, without special attention, a considerable degree of association between the printed letter and the sound it represents. It must be remembered, however, that the special reading disability operates as a distinct obstacle to the association process and we have found it is not safe to assume that when the associative linkages are established in one direction they will also be operative in the other. Thus a child may be able to give promptly the sound equivalent of each letter as it is presented visually and yet be quite unable to give the name of the letter or to produce its graphic form when its sound is presented verbally. Since the reading disability cases without exception are poor spellers it has proved advisable to make sure of all of the usable linkages between vision, audition and kinaesthesis while the reading retraining is under way. It has been our experience that if this be not done reading may advance fairly successfully but spelling will make almost no headway or, as in one striking case, oral spelling may be fairly well acquired but written spelling may remain extremely faulty. This was the case of a young girl who had led her class in spelling in Texas but on moving to Iowa was failing consistently in this subject. On inquiry it was found that in Texas the spelling lessons were always recited aloud while in Iowa lists of words were dictated to be written. The child had not formed a prompt and facile association between the letter name and its graphic form, and while she had no writing disorder her attempts at written spelling were filled with errors of substitution and omission.

Spelling in our experience has been much more difficult of acquisition than reading and much more resistant to special retraining procedures. This can be readily understood when we appreciate that a much less exact mnemonic pattern is necessary for recognition than for recall. Misspelled words will often be read by a poor speller without cognizance of the error, or more frequently the child will say that the word does not look quite right although he is unable to see what is wrong with it. Because of this lack of precision in visual recall of a word it is important to make use of the auditory patterns by means of phonetic dissection as a guide to spelling and to make sure that careful auditory discrimination between closely similar sounds be well established. The short sounds of the vowels, notably $\breve{a}$, $\breve{e}$, and $\breve{i}$, are very apt to be poorly differentiated in the speech of the average child and substitution of one of these sounds for another is frequent. Especial attention should therefore be given to the clear differential enunciation of all of the phonetic units. Errors in the pronunciation of the sounds may make relatively little trouble in reading since a word bearing a compromise sound or even a true substitution of one short vowel for another is often still sufficiently close to the auditory memory of it to bring recognition, but in spelling, of course, such substitutions constitute glaring errors. In English spelling, the problem is further complicated by the fact that a given phonetic unit may often be represented in several ways. It is important therefore for the child to learn that the long sound of *a,* for example, may be designated by *a, ay, ai, ea, eigh,* etc., and practice in telling how many ways we can indicate the *ā* sound is valuable both for reading and for spelling. Unfortunately for these children, the correct choice usually rests on visual familiarity with the word and, since it is in this field that their handicap lies, even with intensive effort on the part of both teacher and pupil, spelling usually lags behind reading by one or more grades.

Phonetic analysis or sound dissection of words which are familiar by ear and accurately spoken but are misspelled in the pupil's oral or written work has frequently proved serviceable in correcting certain types of errors. This often proves to be almost as difficult a procedure for the child at first as is the opposite process of phonetic synthesis or sound blending for the construction of words from their phonetic units as described above. The spoken word has been acquired in both the auditory memory and in the speech mechanism as a unit and not a blend of its parts and often the child is completely at sea at first as to how to approach the dissection. Occasionally even the breaking up of long words into syllables is difficult or impossible although this seems to be more readily learned than the further step of analyzing the syllables themselves into sounds. This approach to the use of the auditory memory of words as an aid to spelling has been of special value in correcting two outstanding types of errors in spelling—omissions of letters and distorted order in assembling the proper letters. Accuracy of speech is naturally of cardinal importance for this purpose. If sounds are omitted or slurred or improperly differentiated in the child's own speech, this is strongly reflected in the spelling of those who do not have an accurate visual recall of the word's appearance. When, for example, such a boy speaks of the "sopperntendent" of his school, he is apt to spell it likewise. Obviously these processes interact and in those words in which the correct spelling has been acquired there is usually a more accurate spoken reproduction although older patterns of slovenly pronunciation may remain, especially in propositional speech, despite knowledge of the spelling of the word. In many cases, a campaign of speech training for accurate and clear enunciation is indicated. When there is not too great a degree of mispronunciation the child may be taught to take apart the blended word into its constituent phonetic units and to name and write each unit as it is isolated. In those children in whom a direct association has been established between the sound of the letter and its graphic reproduction the step of naming is unnecessary and the child separates the phonetic units and writes a symbol for each. Many children, however, have been so thoroughly trained to link the written form of the letter with its name that it is necessary for them, after dissection of the blend into its components, to assign a letter name to each sound so isolated and then to write the corresponding letter. Our experience here has again emphasized the fact that each linkage of the association process must be checked before it can be trusted. Thus it is not uncommon to find a child who, while spelling a word aloud and writing it at the same time, will give the name of the correct letter and yet produce on the paper an entirely different one.

With the severe strephosymbolics who have spent two or three years in school without progress in learning to read there is often a considerable emotional reaction to the failure and an obvious desire to master, at once, this topic in which their classmates have so rapidly outstripped them, and this has naturally raised the question as to how early in the course of the retraining narrative reading may be introduced. In our experience this has generally been unprofitable until the phonetic foundation is secure and the child has begun to learn to blend successfully so that he can see for himself that there is a way to find out what a word "says" even if he does not recall it from its visual presentation. There will be variations here, of course, dependent on many extrinsic influences, but as a rule those children who have experienced several years of exposure to reading with little or no profit are easily intrigued with the fact that this new task is something in which they are not completely "stymied" but in which day to day progress is obvious to them. When carefully encouraged it is thus usually possible to maintain interest and co-operation until such time as actual reading can be begun. One difficulty is often encountered here which is troublesome to overcome, and that is that during the two or three years in which the child has been completely blocked in reading his interests have been expanding at a normal rate so that one is faced with a boy who can be interested only in fourth grade reading material, for example, and yet whose technical skill in reading would limit him to stories of "the little red hen." This not infrequently offers a real challenge to the teacher to find or devise material with a very simple vocabulary and yet with a sufficiently interesting content so that the child is not disheartened by the "babyishness" of the reading on which he must practice. One danger which arises here and which the teacher must be prepared to combat is that the child, stimulated by his success in mastering the phonetic work, may expect too rapid progress in narrative reading and may go through a period of discouragement as he finds that "sounding out," while enabling the reading of individual words, is a very slow process until considerable practice has ultimately fixed the majority of the more frequently encountered words so that they are recognized at sight or can be sounded out so rapidly as to bring almost instant recognition. During this stage of the retraining, the maintenance of the child's morale is extremely important and often presents a problem challenging the ingenuity of the teacher. One measure with which we have experimented to meet this situation is to have the child read part of the story and then to have the teacher read aloud for a time to maintain the interest in the content. It is important, however, to hold the pupil to high standards of accuracy in all of his attempts at oral reading, aiding him only with the words which he is not yet prepared to master by the phonetic approach, in order to prevent a return to earlier habits of guessing or approximation.

In addition to the relief from emotional stress which comes with successful progress in the new way of learning to read, a not unimportant by-product is the change in ease with which the attention can be held and the disappearance of a characteristic motor unrest which is seen in many of these non-readers. With a number of our cases of strephosymbolia the question has been seriously raised by teachers or parents as to whether the whole of their failure in reading might not be caused by a fundamental defect in the attention. This question arises because of their marked distractibility and their tendency to be constantly squirming or wriggling in their chair when confronted with the—for them—impossible task of recognizing words at sight, although they may work with considerable concentration upon other tasks not involving reading. The initiation of phonetic training—a task which can be mastered—often brings a change in these two factors which is little short of miraculous. The child is not only able but willing to sit quietly through a fairly long drill period with excellent attention, and indeed as progress begins to be obvious the attention is often exceptionally well maintained.

No fixed program has been adopted as to the amount of time to be spent on the phonetic drills. As a general rule, however, it has proved advisable to devote not less than one half hour nor more than one hour daily to this work and even this may be cut into several shorter sessions or divided between time spent on giving the phonetic equivalents for the letter cards and in writing letters from dictation of their sounds, etc.

When possible it has seemed wise to have the remedial work incorporated as part of the school day and carried on during the time when the child would otherwise be unprofitably occupied in the regular reading class. This obviates any feeling on the part of the child that he is being punished for failure in reading by having to work after school or during a period which is playtime for the other pupils. Since most of the strephosymbolics have a good auditory memory it has proven valuable at times to offer oral instruction in those subjects which are being covered by the rest of the class and which require reading, such as geography. It is also important at this stage that all of the child's teachers understand his limitations so that he may not be retarded in his learning of arithmetic, for example, by his inability to read the problems for himself, or by reversals in the putting down of a sum correctly added as when 7 + 5 are written as 21 although the child was thinking 12, or by difficulties arising through inconsistency in the direction of carrying or borrowing.

One query which recurs in the discussion of retraining programs is that of how long special work will have to be continued, and to this no definite answer can be given. It is obvious, however, that no miracle such as learning to read fluently in a few weeks or months can be expected and that the program should be planned looking toward two or three years of more or less individualized help with a gradual change in the nature of the remedial work as the child's skills increase and as advances in school grade alter the demands on him.

It will be apparent from the foregoing description of the methods which we have found most successful in retraining children with a severe degree of strephosymbolia that the procedures can only be carried out as a highly individualized program, that is, that the teacher must be prepared to work alone with the child, and this has been found to apply also to those with less extreme degrees of severity who have been overlooked or uncared for during the first years of their schooling, so that there is a striking deficit in both their reading ability and their reading experience. When, however, children who show only mild degrees of the disability are considered, it is pertinent to inquire whether or not treatment in groups may be practicable. One experiment in which these milder cases were segregated from the bulk of the class in the first grade and trained by the phonetic method has been tried and gives promise of considerable success.

For those pupils who, in spite of a moderate handicap in reading, have advanced into the upper grades of grammar school or into junior high school before any effort has been made to correct their disability, as well as for those who have successfully completed the earlier stages of remedial work, oral reading takes an increasingly prominent place in the retraining program. This has usually been dropped out of the school curriculum before these higher grades are reached and tests of the child's ability in this will frequently demonstrate that he has been reading to himself with only an approximation of the correct word sounds and with slurring or omission of many new and difficult words, guessing at the meaning of many of them from the context. If his disability be not severe and he has a good intelligence, he may even be able to obtain passable scores for his age on tests of silent reading comprehension, but he is often unable to make any headway with new or difficult subject material. This sort of reading does not enable him to store memories of words sufficiently clearly to be serviceable in his own speech or writing and he is often at a loss in following some grammatical constructions and in understanding reading material in which practically every word must be grasped for adequate comprehension such as is apt to be demanded of him in his courses in science and mathematics. In such cases, oral reading brings to light many deficiencies in phonetic associations and offers an opportunity to discuss exact word meanings and choices. Reading aloud with emphasis on correct pronunciation and some attention to the construction of exceptional words may also serve as a direct aid to spelling which, in these children, usually lags considerably behind their ability in silent reading comprehension and is much more apt to be found on a level with their ability in oral reading. Study of phonetic choices, word families, spelling rules, prefixes and suffixes, simple derivations and the requirements of grammatical construction have been found profitable at this age.

Unless there be a complicating or associated *motor* disorder such as an agraphia or a speech defect, the problem of handedness is not important in cases of the reading disability. We have found no evidence to show that conversion of a naturally left-handed child to the right-handed pattern plays any part in the genesis of this syndrome and we have also found extreme degrees of strephosymbolia in clear cut dextrals as well as clear cut sinistrals. Since the difficulty can be so clearly related to the sensory cortices there seems to be no good reason for interfering with any pattern of handedness which has been established in the child—be it right or left or converted. Moreover, since the confusions seem to be so clearly referable to the process of recall rather than that of sensation there is, on theoretical grounds at least, no reason to believe that measures aimed at changing the eyedness or those intended to train the eye movements will be particularly profitable, although of course errors in refraction should be corrected with glasses whenever indicated.

One urgent practical question arises in many of these cases and that is, "How far is it justifiable to continue the special training in a particular child?" If the disability be severe or if it has been overlooked for several years, the retraining, to be successful, must be carried out on an individual basis, as has been pointed out, and progress at first is often quite slow. As a consequence, it is a costly form of education and external considerations must be evaluated in determining its practicability in a given case. Here the general intellectual level of the family from which the child comes as well as their economic status must be considered. The relative degree of disability which the child exhibits and his probable latent intelligence, together with his own vocational interests, are also factors of importance in such a decision. However, it must be remembered that reading and writing, while not essential in all trades, are an important part of the equipment in any, and that advancement in almost any occupation will depend in part at least on the possession of at least a reasonable amount of skill with these two fundamental intellectual tools. Moreover, when we see pupils with the reading disability repeating year after year of schooling, the question may well be raised as to whether the tutoring required to give such a child a start in reading might not prove less costly in the long run to both parent and school than are the many repetitions.

It may be noted that the methods recommended here are diametrically opposed to those which are currently in use in many schools. There has been in recent years a striking swing toward the use of the sight or flash-card method of teaching reading and away from the use of phonetics. The writer is not in a position to offer an opinion as to the efficacy of either of these methods as a general school procedure but their effect on children suffering from varying degrees of strephosymbolia has come under his immediate attention and he feels that there can be no doubt that the use of the popular flash method of teaching reading is a definite obstacle to children who suffer from any measure of this disability. We have no new numerical data to offer here since our work recently has dealt exclusively with referred cases and we have made no general surveys of the number of cases of the reading disabilities in schools using different methods. At an earlier period, however, some such surveys were undertaken in Iowa and they indicated strongly that where the sight or flash-card method of teaching reading was exclusively used, the number of reading disability cases was increased by three times that found in schools which used phonetic training for those children who did not rapidly progress by the flash-card method. As a further measure of the comparative efficiency of these two methods of teaching when dealing with a case of specific reading disability, it may be said that we have retrained a number of children who had not progressed beyond first grade reading skills after having spent three or four years in schools where the sight method was used exclusively, and have been able to advance them by two or more reading grades in one academic year by the application of the phonetic method. This has also been true in many cases in which the school program had been previously supplemented by intensive individual work but with no phonetic training or at best very inadequate attempts along these lines. It may also be noted in passing that the great majority of the children whom we have seen have not shown any lack of desire to learn to read although they may have been prevented from obtaining any profit or pleasure from efforts to read by themselves in the past because of their very deficient skills. Indeed, a reading disability may be suspected whenever a child does not occasionally turn to reading for pastime and, conversely, when remedial reading training has been successful in supplying the child with a usable skill, his interest in reading will usually develop spontaneously and he will commence at once to make up for lost time.

It would obviously be advantageous, were it possible, to select those children who have a strephosymbolic tendency at the time of their entry into school, or before, and thus build a preventive program rather than to await the advent of the trouble and then institute *re*training. Practically all children, however, show a tendency to confusion of reversible letters and to occasional sinistrad reading of reversible words, and no means have yet been devised which will indicate whether these ambivalent tendencies in visual recall will persist and make trouble or whether they will rapidly disappear. We cannot yet therefore make a se-

Problems in Children

lection for preventive treatment but there are certain children who might be said to be under suspicion as potential reading disability cases. These include the stutterers whose impediment began with their earliest speech, children with difficulty in understanding the spoken word, the apraxics, and those who have been very late in making a choice of a master hand. As far as our observations go at present those with good understanding of the speech of others but who are slow in developing their own speech are less apt to encounter trouble with reading than is the case with the other groups mentioned. A family history of left-handedness or of the occurrence of other cases of developmental language disorders should put us on guard for a reading disability, but is of no import as to the outlook in any particular child. Obviously, however, the earlier special measures are adopted for children with special needs, the greater will be the chance of ultimate success, and we feel that no child with average intelligence or better should be allowed to continue into his second year of schooling, if there be tangible evidence of a reading difficulty, without an analysis to determine whether or not he be of the strephosymbolic group so that special measures may be instituted, when indicated, before he suffers the emotional disorders and language deficits which are usually cumulative from this time on.

In the chapter dealing with the various syndromes met in children, we have spoken of cases first seen after they have reached the late years of the secondary schools or the early years of college as cases exhibiting the residuals of a mild strephosymbolia, and almost without exception this is warranted from the standpoint of their educational history since the record of their early school years gives evidence of marked delay in learning to read and characteristic persistent difficulty with spelling. When viewed, however, from the symptomatology as seen in later years, the disorder is often not so much that of recognition of words as it is that of the comprehension of the meaning of series of words forming sentences and paragraphs. Lack of facility in written expression also marks some of these cases and the two syndromes might therefore be better considered as the counterpart in the reading sphere of Kleist's "sentence deafness" and "sentence muteness" with their characteristic paragrammatic and agrammatic defects respectively. Only a very few of our cases of typical strephosymbolics, who were recognized as such at an early stage of their education and who have been retrained in reading, have as yet progressed as far as college, and the number of those who have been studied for the first time after their entry into college is also comparatively small. Retraining experiments are under way in some such cases and with promise of real betterment, but the series is too restricted in number to permit of an expression regarding the best methods of treatment. Our experiments to date have followed the simple plan of a very careful analysis of the language function from both the oral and visual standpoint and the institution of measures aimed at the correction of the more patent shortcomings. This must obviously be a highly individualized program and since it leads directly into questions of nicety of word discrimination, of etymology and of syntax, as well as the ability to select the significant concepts from a paragraph or a chapter, it requires tutors with a considerable educational background of their own. One very serviceable point, however, should be mentioned, and that is that the same student who may fail sadly to grasp the meaning of material which he reads for himself, may be able to understand quite well the same material read aloud to him by someone else. One pupil who had been dropped from college for failure in the midyear examinations of his freshman year was reinstated provisionally under an oral tutorial program and was able to carry his work successfully in this manner and has since been graduated. The whole problem of these older patients, however, is still in a highly experimental stage and forms one of the frontiers for further research.

2. Developmental Agraphia

In those children who have encountered especial difficulty in learning to write either with serviceable speed or acceptable legibility, tests of skill in the two hands and a history of handedness development in childhood are of utmost importance since here we meet many problems primarily motor in nature.

A considerable number of those who have trouble learning to write are frank left-handers who have been taught from the beginning to use their right hands for writing. Obviously many natural sinistrals have acquired a legible and rapid writing with the right hand but there are others in whom speed or legibility has suffered by this enforced shift and still others who write well and rapidly with the right hand but in whom the threshold of fatigue is low or who find that the mechanics of right-hand writing distracts them to some degree from the content of their compositions. There seems to be no age limit beyond which retraining of the left hand for writing cannot be fairly easily accomplished in strongly left-sided individuals. For the right-handed adult, learning to use the left hand for writing is arduous, but it is often surprising how quickly and easily this skill can be acquired even in adult life by a native sinistral. We have recommended a shift to the naturally preferred left hand, with successful results, to several boys in their "teens" and to one college graduate. The latter was strongly left-sided in everything except writing in which use of the right hand had been enforced from the beginning. He was ambitious to study medicine but had serious misgivings as to its advisability because of the troubles that he had encountered in written work in college and because he felt that the large amount of note taking and written examinations in medical school might prove too much for him. Learning to write with the left hand proved very easy for him and its use lessened fatigue and the tendency to finger cramps strikingly, and gave him at least a subjective feeling of much greater ease of expression in written work. Following this shift he entered medical school and is competing there successfully.

Although the experience of the examiner plays some part in determining when a shift to the left hand in such individuals should be recommended, there are no tests or criteria which can be trusted here because of the great variability in the degree of left-hand skill in native sinistrals, and our approach to this problem has been an experimental one. When the history of left-handedness from early infancy is clear and when the left is preferred in other activities than writing and

Problems in Children

when motor tests show an equivalent or superior skill in finer movements, other than writing, with the left hand, we have advised left-hand writing as a trial procedure for a few months. If in that time the left has not acquired a writing ability equal to or better than that previously attained by the right, the attempt is discontinued. No estimate of the exact time required to learn to write with the left hand can safely be made.

It cannot always be assumed that the left-handed child should be taught to write with the left hand since in some whom we have studied, in spite of marked superiority in all other motor acts on the left, writing proved very laborious and cramped and in a few instances of this type we have recommended a shift to the right hand for writing only, with a subsequent marked improvement in both speed and quality of the product. Such cases illustrate clearly the highly individual character of each writing problem and certain factors observed in these cases suggest that motor facilities alone do not always determine optimum usage but that sensory factors probably also are operative in the acquisition of writing.

As mentioned in the chapter on diagnosis a proper position of the paper and hand will greatly facilitate the acquisition of left-hand writing both in the case of left-handed children who are just learning to write and in the mistrained left-handers who are experimenting with a shift. The proper position of the paper is the exact mirror opposite of that employed for right-handed children, that is, with the top of the sheet inclined toward the *right*. This is of so much importance as a training factor that an illustration of the exact position is given here. (Figure 24) Careful attention to this will permit the child to follow easily across the page without contortion and without dragging his hand through the ink of freshly written lines.

A second factor which is frequently of considerable aid to the left-handed writer is the determination of the easiest and most natural slant and this applies often to right-handed patients also. As a general rule,

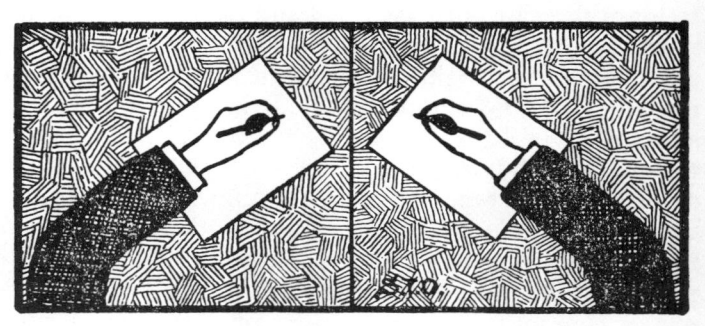

FIGURE 24. *A sketch to show the corresponding positions of the paper and hand for left- and right-handed writers.*

the right-handed person tends to slant his letters with their top toward the right but this is not consistent and not a few right-handed writers develop a "backhand" or slant toward the left. Conversely, with the left-handers a backhand writing seems somewhat more common but again this is not always so and it has been found very helpful to determine the slant in which strokes and letter forms can be most easily made. Observations of the natural inclination are made from samples of writing, and to further test this we ask the patient to draw rapidly a series of short lines parallel to each other in the forward slant, in the vertical and in the backhand direction. Similar tests using loops such as those that form parts of letters are also employed and for the older children paper ruled with ink in parallel lines in each of the three slants can be inserted under a thin sheet of paper and experiments in writing following each of the slants are then made. Frequently a strong preference for one or the other pattern will be immediately apparent and it has been found profitable to follow this choice in subsequent training.

While abnormal difficulty in writing is fairly frequently encountered in mistrained and masked left-handers, it is by no means limited to them. It occurs not infrequently in those children who have been slow to choose either hand as a master and in the apraxic children and also in some who seem to have developed early a marked preference for right-sidedness in hand, eye and foot. One very serviceable procedure which we have used with some of the poor writers is that of teaching the child to produce the letter from its "feel" or kinaesthetic pattern rather than by visual guidance. For this purpose the child learns to draw the letter form from a pattern set at a distance and with the paper on which he is writing hidden by a cardboard shield. Once the patterns have been established, practice in this may be carried out with the eyes closed or even blindfolded. The obvious purpose of this method is to train the kinaesthetic patterns so that the hand will more or less automatically produce the letter form without visual control much as the practiced typist finds the proper keys while her eyes follow a manuscript. One noticeable result of practice of this sort is often an immediate relief from the cramped position of the hand and "pencil squeezing" which were apparent before it was instituted. This method proved of value in the retraining of the girl who showed a latent mirror-writing skill and whose product is shown in Figure 17. The patient whose mirror-writing skill is illustrated in Figure 18 was a medical student at the time his disability was studied and no formal retraining was undertaken with him. He was shown, however, that if he inserted a sheet of carbon paper face up beneath the sheet on which he was writing in the mirrored form, it would reproduce the writing in reverse so that he could write in mirror writing on one side of the sheet and turn it over to read it. This was an obvious subterfuge but a serviceable one.

In spite of the employment of the various devices outlined above we have encountered a number of children who progressed very slowly in the acquisition of an acceptable handwriting, and in such cases it may be well to give up the time-consuming writing drills and teach the child to use the typewriter. We have no evidence from our own experiments, however, as to the relative facility with which such children can learn to use this instrument.

In the special writing disability the formation of sequences plays an important part. Many children who can produce each letter symbol quickly and easily in isolation have great trouble in writing words, and this is true whether they be using the cursive or manuscript form. There also is usually much greater difficulty in propositional work than in writing to dictation and this in turn is more difficult than copying. These facts have been considered in planning the school work advised for children who have this handicap as well as in designing the course of their retraining. The first of their practice work has, as a rule, been copying from printed text and only when the mechanics of this have improved considerably have they been asked to write to dictation. We have also advised that these children be excused from all written work if possible in school while the retraining is under way in order that the effect of a careful practice period be not entirely submerged by the need to write under pressure with the rest of the class.

3. Developmental Word Deafness

The number of cases in which word deafness was an outstanding feature and in which we have had an opportunity to undertake experiments in retraining is very small, but the results have been suggestively promising. Starting with the assumption that in this disorder the trouble lay in the recall of sequences of word sounds in the correct time order, comparable to the difficulty in recall of spatial sequences in developmental word blindness, we have undertaken to teach the child orally the separate phonetic units and to purify or correct such as he produced improperly or in confusion and then to proceed through simple blending to short words, at the same time building a visual association of the word with an object of the environment or with a picture to fix its meaning. None of our younger cases in whom we believed word deafness to be a factor has as yet advanced far enough to permit a judicious estimate of the ultimate outcome, although some have made good progress. In two older boys, however, in whom the failure of understanding of spoken words was a confronting symptom, a very considerable response has ensued to this program. In both of these cases the value of clear enunciation, the choice of simple words, short sentences and slow speech on the part of the teacher was very apparent. In one case, when the boy was asked the question, "Did you enjoy camp enough this summer to want to go again?", it was met with a blank expression and elicited no response whatever. When, however, this was broken up into the two queries "Did you like camp?" and "Do you want to go again?", the response to both was instant and enthusiastic. With both of these boys their ability to understand a rapid-fire talker was much less than that when the same requests or commands were given by a slow and careful speaker. The older of these boys was seventeen years old when we first saw him but he had reached only about the second grade level in school. A full-time tutor working under the guidance of the Language Research Unit was provided for him and as far as possible all educational procedures made use of objective tasks or concepts while careful training of the speech by phonetic synthesis was also instituted. When he was first seen, this boy's speech was filled with inaccuracies, clipped words, misuse of words and showed frequent neologisms. During a two-year period of such instruction by a tutor the neologisms and mutilated words completely disappeared, he showed a very marked betterment in his ability to comprehend the speech of others as well as to express himself in comprehensible form and his general educational level was raised by four grades or more.

For those children in whom a true regional deafness involving the frequencies within the speech range exists, the special methods employed by teachers of the deaf are indicated and these will not be reviewed here. A word concerning one adjuvant form of treatment may be offered, however, since some of the older patients of this group have learned to read comparatively well and with these selected cases some improvement in the associated speech defect can be built upon the visual memory of the word structure by careful instruction by a teacher versed in phonetic practices. Thus the knowledge of the spelling of the word can be used to implant in the speech of these patients the presence of a letter sound which they have learned to reproduce by kinaesthetic memory but which they cannot hear either in their own speech or in the speech of others.

4. *Developmental Motor Aphasia*

The children who are very slow in learning to talk and who often show many infantilisms in their speech as well but who have no difficulty in understanding the speech of others have responded to treatment as a rule most encouragingly. In our procedure a careful survey has first been made of the phonetic units which the child can echo after the examiner and where any such units were lacking or faulty they were taught by the methods in common use by teachers of speech. The major difficulty in these cases has been found almost without exception to rest on an inability to blend sounds which can be reproduced in isolation and our experiments have been aimed at teaching the child the simplest sort of blending, consisting at first of only one consonant followed by one vowel until this process has been mastered, when longer sequences are very gradually introduced. For this step we have used both short words and nonsense syllables in order to cover a very wide range of sound blends. Starting with the teaching of whole words, as is so commonly practiced, even though they be short ones, does not seem to be so profitable as this process of beginning a little further back with only two sounds at first and gradually increasing the span. Certainly the initiation of this program should be in the hands of a person experienced in the teaching of speech correction and conversant with the special methods employed in such work. Although later it is probable that the retraining can be carried on by a somewhat less highly trained technical aide, it is nevertheless important that the instructor chosen be someone with clear enunciation and slow, deliberate speech. The propositional element plays a part here comparable to that mentioned in the writing disability and marked defects in this type of speech are to be expected for a considerable period after the child has learned to echo with accuracy and even after he can repeat memorized material without errors. The emphasis in training must in general correspond to these stages of development in the child's speech. The majority of these children are seen at about the age of three or four and frequently the difficulty has improved markedly, either spontaneously or as a result of training, before the child has reached school age. Some of them, however, will enter school before the difficulty has been fully corrected and a moderate easement in the demands for oral recitations is often advisable. A phonetic approach to reading has also proved of value in clearing up residual defects in speech after the child has entered school.

Many of our cases which fall in this group have been children who were also very slow in making a choice of a master hand or who showed marked motor intergrading, and the history of a number who were very "late talkers" has revealed a close relationship in time between a spontaneous betterment in speech and an increasing tendency to selective use of one hand. We have therefore experimented with a program of training to increase the skills and freedom of use of one hand. Obviously, careful motor tests of handedness and eyedness must precede this in order to determine which hand to train, and not infrequently this will lead the examiner into a dilemma which can only be resolved by experiment. A wide variety of games are useful here, both overhand throwing as with a baseball or darts and underhand tossing as with rope rings or quoits, and indoor games such as jack straws, tiddlywinks, etc., also have been employed. Because of the fact that spontaneous improvement is the rule in these cases and because the motor training has been carried out at the same time as specific speech training, it is impossible to say how valuable the hand exercises have been. However, many of these children with delayed speech of the motor type become stutterers when they begin to talk and handedness training has proven its value in some early stutterers, so it would seem to be indicated. Moreover, the practice in a variety of games will do no harm and is often a distinct asset to the child in his athletic competition with his fellows.

Some of the children with delayed speech but good understanding show such extreme degrees of difficulty in learning other movements that they may be classed among the apraxics. With this group progress in learning the speech blends has tended to be very slow. A few cases have been studied in which handedness training contrary to the child's natural bent has been very closely associated in time at least with a speech regression. One such boy who exhibited a decided preference for his left hand had begun to talk fairly freely when rather rigorous right-hand training was instituted by his parents. This was almost immediately followed by a period of complete mutism which did not disappear until training for left-handed superiority was again instituted.

5. Developmental Apraxia

Among the children finding unusual difficulty in learning patterns of movement is to be found an occasional individual who is a shifted left-hander and who never has been successful in acquiring skills on the right although this may be the side used extensively. Where history and motor tests indicate this to be the case a retraining of the left hand may do much to offset the unskillfulness. A much more intricate problem is presented by the majority of apraxic children, however, since their unskillfulness extends to both hands—they are "doubly left-handed" and often amphiocular as well—and no latent abilities are uncovered by tests in either the right or the left side. The number of cases which we have studied in which apraxia was the outstanding symptom is not large and our facilities for extended experiments in training were not of the best but a few observations and results nevertheless seem worthy of record while awaiting the opportunity to

Problems in Children

extend this line of research with additional cases and experiments. Our attention has been directed to attempting to determine very simple patterns of movement over which the child has a reasonable mastery, and gradually combining these simpler patterns into more complex and difficult ones. Here again we have been guided by the belief that it is in such recombinations of simple movements that the crux of the apraxic child's difficulty rests.

At times the motor inaptitude seems to involve movements of the body as a whole including such factors as balance and gait and not merely the more complex movements which underlie manual dexterity. These children are often quite proficient in activities such as swimming and horseback riding where the body is supported without so great a need for equilibration, but the gross movements of the body in such acts as walking, running and jumping are very poorly executed. This was the case with one girl of about six years of age who walked with a very clumsy stride and who could "never walk up stairs without stumbling on at least every other step." She also had tried to learn some very simple dance steps from one of her teachers but her efforts in this were far from a reproduction of the demonstrated pattern. To train the stepping movements for stair climbing, two by ten inch wooden blocks were employed and the child was taught to put only the ball of the foot on the block and then to raise the body enough to bring the toe of the other foot clear when it was swung forward. This was practiced on one foot at a time before a second block was added and progressional alternating steps were permitted. Next, the height of the blocks was increased to four inches and gradually a very satisfactory result was attained on the stairs. It may be remarked in passing that the learning of many of our skilled acts depends on visual observation of the movements of others and that these visual models must then be retranslated into kinaesthetic-motor patterns. With this idea in mind, experiments were tried with the dance steps with both the child and her teacher standing before a large mirror so that the teacher's movements were reflected as on the same side in which the child was attempting to copy them, and this procedure was much more successful than were attempts at vis-à-vis imitation.

It is common to assume that the simple, largely reflex patterns of movement which enter into walking and running, for example, are sufficiently well acquired by the child without training so that in the more difficult sports, such as tennis, attention need be given only to the special instruction for that game and this, of course, is true of most children. In those with a measure of apraxia in their make-up, however, this assumption is not justified and much better headway might be made by spending some time teaching the child how to run and turn and stop without losing balance, before specific training in the sport is begun.

In those apraxic children whose clumsiness is expressed chiefly in learning manual skills, one symptomatic indication would seem to be to raise the level of dexterity in one side above that of the other by games such as those mentioned above, and since no superiority can, as a rule, be demonstrated on either side in these children, we are left with a choice as to which side shall be trained. Under such circumstances our advice has favored the right hand to conform with the

Problems in Children

more generally used pattern of the community at large.

One issue not infrequently raised by parents of these children is that of what their reaction should be toward the excessive awkwardness which leads to spilled food at table, upset milk glasses, etc. It often helps the parent to understand that this condition may be a real disability and not merely excessive carelessness. Obviously, punishment or scolding for such accidents is not just nor does it seem to be efficacious since too much attention paid to the mishaps may increase the difficulty. How this operates is not clear but it seems to be related to the greater trouble inherent in the propositional or effortful element already noted in the writing disability cases and those with a motor speech delay and which comes into its fullest flower in stuttering. Possibly the best attitude for the parents to adopt is that of tolerant amusement toward each episode but with careful observation of the faulty movements, looking toward sympathetic instruction for their correction.

A considerable measure of feeling of inferiority seems to be unavoidable in the apraxics, especially as these children grow to the age when they enter active physical competition where their limitations must be rather piteously exposed. While the acquisition of skills is arduous for the apraxic, almost any technique can be mastered with sufficient application and practice, and sometimes slow but punctilious training in some one sport or manual craft will serve to compensate largely for the more general awkwardness. Thus, in one of the writer's patients, a question about tennis brought up some obviously rather painful recollections of experiences on the court but the child was prompt to volunteer at this stage that she had by persistence learned to sew quite well. She later brought in a sample of her work which showed almost meticulous neatness and accuracy in stitching. Fortunately, many of the apraxic cases are quite successful competitors in their scholastic work and this is frequently a source of satisfaction which serves as a recompense for their failures in athletics and manual work.

6. Stuttering in Childhood

The childhood stutterers for the purpose of this discussion of treatment must be separated into two groups, viz.—those who stutter from the time they first begin to talk and those whose speech is normal until the sixth to eighth year. In the younger group it is exceedingly important to determine whether a shift of handedness away from the natural inclination has taken place or is under way. Motor tests as well as very careful inquiry into the history is essential here. If the child has been shifted and if the motor patterns are good on the abandoned side, retraining of all unilateral activities in the native hand is always worth the experiment and is often accompanied by a fairly prompt cessation of the stuttering. One of the writer's patients—a boy of three—had stuttered only a few weeks when he was first examined. When the parents were questioned as to his handedness, the mother was sure he was right-handed although the father—questioned separately—described him as "fifty-fifty." Tests and brief observations suggested a strong leaning toward the left hand and the parents were advised to take him home for a week and observe him carefully from this standpoint. At the end of that period, they reported that he used his left hand in all but three activities and in these he was being trained to use his right. These were, however, among the most difficult patterns that he was acquiring at that time. A reversal of these training procedures, that is, a free use of the left hand for all one-sided acts, was followed by a complete disappearance of the stuttering within a few weeks.

Unfortunately such cases as that above quoted have given rise to the frequently heard statement that all stutterers should have been left-handed and ought to be so trained. This rests on a very superficial comprehension of the complexities of the problem of cerebral dominance and of the potential sources of difficulty. In many of our cases there is no superiority of the left hand and no indication of an enforced change from the native pattern. Many of them are marked motor intergrades with no clear preference for either hand, but some—and this applies particularly to those with a very strong hereditary lading toward stuttering—are as clearly as we can determine exclusively right-sided from the beginning.

In those children in whom there is a strong mixture of right- and left-side patterns we have tried to increase the lead of one side or the other by the same training measures which have been described in connection with motor speech delay. In the stutterers this seems to be somewhat more productive than in those children whose speech is late in developing.

In many of this group of younger stutterers and particularly in those who have been slow in learning to speak at all, there are phonetic errors complicating the picture. This varies all the way from one or two infantilisms to imperfections in almost all of the speech sounds. When this is true, accurate phonetic training by standard methods is indicated as the first measure of treatment. From this starting point, practice in blending of the units, starting with very short series and gradually increasing the length of the letter groups has been used with considerable success. Where the handedness is clear and the child is old enough, a beginning may be made in the building of associations between the sound of a letter and its written form. This may serve a double purpose since many of these early stutterers are prone to letter reversals and confusions and not a few of them prove to be typical cases of strephosymbolia by the time they encounter reading.

In the six- to eight-year-old group of stutterers there has usually been a history of normal development and use of speech until this critical period is reached. The chief problem of handedness which has been encountered here is that of right-handed training in writing in a left-handed child or one who is a marked intergrade but with considerable latent skill on the left. Where this is occurring, a retraining of the writing in the correct left-hand pattern is frequently sufficient to cure the stuttering without other measures. In a good many cases, however, the issue cannot be so clearly drawn as this and it is frequently difficult to decide which hand should be used in writing. As with the younger group, training to increase the superiority of the master hand has seemed to be of value, although not quite so markedly so. Where phonetic defects exist, careful training should be instituted to correct the errors and this should be followed by practice in sound blending. The children of this group have not in our experience had much strephosymbolia but they are very prone to have a great deal of trouble with their handwriting, often sufficient to warrant the diagnosis of a developmental motor agraphia. When this occurs, the special methods described under that title have been applied.

When writing has been acquired with moderate speed and skill it can be used to advantage as a training procedure for the stutterer. While the younger group of stutterers are apt to have serious difficulty with reading, the older ones usually learn to comprehend their reading material readily, but oral reading is very difficult because of stuttering in the words being read. In these "reading stutterers" the episodes occur almost exclusively on the initial sounds of the words they are reading and if such a child traces the initial letter of each word with a pencil while he is reading it, he is able to read with few or no stuttering blocks. This "pencil facilitation" for oral reading is at first applied to the initial letter of every word and this makes for a slow, staccato delivery. After some practice in reading by this method, initialing every word, it is usually possible to reduce the use of the pencil to tracing the initials of only every second or third word or only the initial of the first word of a phrase or sentence, until gradually the penciling can be omitted or used only for long or unfamiliar words. It is important in this procedure that the pencil be in motion, tracing the letter, before the speech effort is initiated. If speaking begins first, the penciling will not help. Gradually by this procedure it has been possible in a number of cases to free the reading from stuttering blocks entirely but the amount of "carry over" which occurs into propositional speech is variable. In some cases, no further training of the speech was necessary. Much more frequently, however, the defect remains with little or no improvement in propositional speech even after reading has responded. It is possible to apply the pencil facilitation to propositional speech also, but this is a difficult technique for a child to master and as a rule practice in blending seems to have been equally profitable.

The attitude of the young stutterer is often an obstacle to treatment—he does not permit his handicap to interfere with his activities as a rule and is apt to be either mildly unco-operative or actively resentful of the time asked of him for the training procedures. This frequently is a decisive challenge to the teacher who is working with him and the success with which it is met may determine the outcome of the program to a considerable extent. Home discipline of the young stutterer is important and should be carried out as it would be for a normal child. Too frequently we meet the stuttering child whose difficulty has been blamed on that nebulous quality known as "nervousness," who has been allowed to escape all discipline and who consequently is too poorly controlled to be examined properly or to co-operate in any form of retraining.

It is wise to avoid all strong competition in speech —particularly of the argumentative type—for the stutterer both at home, in school and as far as possible on the playground. The demands for oral responses in school should be reduced to the minimum acceptable or if possible eliminated entirely during the training period and the child should be given the opportunity of writing his recitations or of reciting in private to the teacher. The fact that propositional speech suffers most in the stutterer and that repetitive speech is frequently free of blocks can often be capitalized by permitting the child to commit to memory those recitations from which he should not be excused. Such a child can also often take his share in school plays and other special programs if his part be learned by heart.

The emotional factors must also be carefully studied and the child must be guided through this period to prevent the development of the personality disorders which form so prominent a feature in the case of adult stutterers. The six- to eight-year-old stutterers, and this applies with equal force to the reading and writing disability cases, are old enough and intelligent enough usually to understand a simply phrased explanation of the probable organic genesis of their trouble. They are usually interested in the story of how only one side of the brain works in the language function and intrigued with the idea that the two halves of their brain may be "squabbling over which is to be the boss" and pleased when it is possible to tell them, as it frequently is on the basis of intelligence tests, that their brains are better than average but not working just right for the particular subject in which they have met trouble. This sort of an understanding of how his difficulty may have arisen will often go a long way toward preventing the child from falling back later on explanations based on emotional instability, "nervousness," undue fears or lack of self-confidence which in themselves are not entirely emotionally acceptable and which often seem to operate as a vicious circle.

An even more complete explanation to the parents and to the teachers of the specific nature of all of these difficulties is of prime importance in treatment of the child since the school failures have all too often been interpreted as due to some degree of mental defect or to defective attention or to laziness or to poor training, and frequently with an implication of blame which may very easily foster an unwarranted feeling of guilt in the child or the parent or both.

CONCLUSION

The view here presented that many of the delays and defects in development of the language function may arise from a deviation in the process of establishing unilateral brain superiority in individual areas, while taking account of the hereditary facts, brings with it the conviction that such disorders should respond to specific training if we become sufficiently keen in our diagnosis and if we prove ourselves clever enough to devise the proper training methods to meet the needs of each particular case.

Glossary

A GLOSSARY OF SOME TECHNICAL TERMS AS THEY ARE USED IN THIS VOLUME

ACTION CURRENT—An electric current occurring during action of a nerve or muscle.

AGE—1. *Chronological*—Age in years and months as usually calculated.

2. *Mental*—A rating, expressed in years and months, of the development of the intelligence of an individual as measured by certain standardized tests.

AGENETIC—Defective development—as applied to the brain, a failure in growth of certain parts of the brain.

AGNOSIA—Loss of the power to recognize the import of sensations. The varieties correspond with the several senses and are distinguished as auditory, visual, gustatory, tactile, etc. Visual agnosia is equivalent to mind-blindness, auditory to mind-deafness. *Astereognosis* is a special form of this condition in which there is loss of ability to recognize objects by handling them without seeing them.

AGRAMMATISM—Inability to utter words in their correct sequences; impairment of the power to speak grammatically and syntactically due to brain injury or brain disease.

AGRAPHIA—1. *Acquired*—Loss of a previous ability to write resulting from brain injury or brain disease.

2. *Developmental (Congenital)*—Unusual difficulty in learning to write which is out of harmony with the other intellectual accomplishments and manual skills of the individual.

ALEXIA—1. *Acquired*—Loss of a previous skill in reading which follows disease or damage to certain parts of the brain.

Developmental (Congenital)—Inability to learn to read with the rapidity and skill which would be expected from the individual's mental age and achievements in other subjects.

AMBILEVOUS—Poor in manual dexterity with both hands; "doubly left-handed." *cf.* Ambidextrous.

AMBIVALENCE (a. Ambivalent)—Having equal power in two contrary directions.

AMNESIA—Loss of memory.

AMPHIOCULARITY (a. Amphiocular)—Using either eye for sighting without consistent preference. *See* Master Eye.

ANGULAR GYRUS—*See* Gyrus.

ANTITROPE (a. Antitropic)—Alike except for opposite orientation, as, for example, a pair of gloves.

APHASIA (a. Aphasic)—1. *Acquired*—A loss in the power of expression by speech, writing or signs or of comprehending spoken or written language, due to injury or disease of the brain centers.

2. *Developmental (Congenital)*—A failure in development of speech or speech understanding which is not the result of deafness or of defect in the peripheral speech mechanism.

APRAXIA (a. Apraxic)—1. *Acquired*—The loss, as a result of injury or disease of parts of the brain, of previously acquired skilled acts, not dependent on paralysis.

2. *Developmental (Congenital)*—A failure in development of normal skills—abnormal clumsiness.

AREA (As applied to the brain)—Area may designate an anatomical region of the brain, as when we speak of the frontal area, or it may be restricted to parts of the

Glossary

brain which have a common function as in the term *motor area* (*q.v.*) or it may be used in describing a part of the brain which has a characteristic microscopic structure such as the *area striata* (*q.v.*).

Area, Motor—That part of the brain cortex in which lie the giant nerve cells which are in direct command of voluntary motion and whose destruction results in paralysis of voluntary motion, but without loss of reflex or involuntary movements.

Area Striata—That part of the brain cortex which is characterized by a heavy band of nerve fibers not found elsewhere so strongly developed. The white line formed by these fibers is prominent enough to be seen by the naked eye, and the cortex so marked is the terminus of the nerve paths coming from the eyes and forms an important part of the visual center of the brain.

ARRIVAL PLATFORM—That part of the brain cortex to which the nerve fibers carrying a given sensation are distributed. Thus we recognize an arrival platform for vision, for audition, etc. As a rule the microscopic structure of these areas is quite different from those surrounding them. *See* Area Striata.

ASSOCIATION—The process by which a stimulus becomes connected with previous experiences or other stimuli. *Associative linkages*—the connection existing in memory between two associated stimuli.

AUDIOGRAM—*See* Audiometer.

AUDIOMETER—A device to test the power of hearing. As generally used this instrument can be used not only to test hearing in general but to compare the acuity for each of a number of pitches, and the record made from such a test of a considerable pitch range in a given individual is called an *Audiometer-Curve* or simply an *Audiogram*.

BASE DEAFNESS—*See* Deafness.

BLEND, PHONETIC—The fusion of individual letter sounds as they are combined in ordinary speech.

BLINDNESS—1. *Cortical-Blindness*—Loss of vision resulting from destruction of the visual center (arrival platform) in the brain, but without disease or disorder of the eyes or optic nerves.

2. *Mind-Blindness* (*Visual Agnosia*)—Loss of the ability to recognize objects by sight although they are still seen.

3. *Word-Blindness*—(a) Acquired—Loss of the ability to recognize the meanings of printed or written words.

(b) Developmental (Congenital)—Inability in learning to read which is out of harmony with the individual's general intelligence and ability to learn by other channels.

BRAIN CENTER—A part of the brain which is devoted to one function, as, for example, the *motor center*. *See* Area.

CEREBRAL—Pertaining to the cerebrum or main portion of the brain.

CEREBRAL DOMINANCE—*See* Dominance.

CEREBRAL LOCALIZATION—The study of the part which various brain areas play in its functions.

CLINICAL—The study of the living patient (literally at the bedside) as contrasted with autopsy and laboratory studies.

CLONIC SPASM—*See* Spasm.

CONGENITAL—Belonging to one from birth, as differentiated from *acquired* which is the result of some influence acting after birth.

CONVOLUTIONS, BRAIN—*See* Gyrus.

CORTEX, BRAIN (pl. Cortices, a. Cortical)—The outer surface of the brain which contains the nerve cells and

Glossary

most of their inter-connections. It is grayish in color as compared to the underlying white matter which contains no nerve cells and which is made up almost entirely of nerve fibers connecting various areas. It is the cortex which is referred to as the "gray matter" of the brain. The various cortices may be referred to according to their function, as, for example, *the motor cortex,* or by anatomical location as in the *parieto-occipital cortex.*

DEAFNESS—1. *Cortical-Deafness*—Loss of hearing as a result of destruction of the auditory arrival platforms but with no disease of the ears or auditory nerves.
2. *Mind-Deafness (Auditory Agnosia)*—Loss of the ability to understand the meaning of sounds of the environment although they are heard.
3. *Word-Deafness*—(a) Acquired—Loss of the ability to understand the spoken word.
    (b) Developmental (Congenital)—Difficulty in learning to understand spoken words.
4. *Regional Deafness*—Lowered acuity of hearing in a part only of the normal range of pitch. This may include chiefly the lower range when it is called *bass deafness,* but more commonly the higher range is affected, resulting in *high-frequency deafness.*
5. *Peripheral Deafness*—Deafness due to disease of the ear or auditory nerve as contrasted with that due to brain lesions as described above.

DEMENTIA—A degradation from a previously acquired mental level.

DEVELOPMENTAL—Incidental to growth. As used in this volume in connection with the various language disorders this term is intended to include intrinsic factors—both hereditary and congenital, and extrinsic influences of the environment, such as training, which play a part in the development and evolution of the language faculty in the individual, thus giving a somewhat broader range to the expression *developmental alexia,* for example, than was true of its predecessor *congenital alexia.* The *developmental disorders of language* are those in which there is exhibited a specific difficulty in acquisition or learning as contrasted to the *acquired* in which there is a loss of a previously acquired skill.

DEXTRAD—Toward the right side or hand or in the right-hand direction.

DEXTRAL—Right. Also used as an abbreviation for a right-handed person.

DIGRAPH—A group of two letters representing a single speech sound, as, for example, *th.*

DIPHTHONG—A union of two vowels forming a compound sound such as *oy.* Where two vowels represent one sound as in *ea* they constitute, strictly speaking, a digraph, and are sometimes called *improper diphthongs.*

DOMINANCE (a. Dominant)—1. *Cerebral Dominance.* When used by physiologists without further qualification this refers to the increasingly important role played by the cerebral cortex, as the animal scale is ascended, in controlling and integrating the activities of the lower nervous centers such, for example, as the cerebellum and the spinal cord.

2. *Unilateral Cerebral Dominance.* When used with this qualifying adjective the expression refers to the concentration of functional control of language in one half of the brain such as is revealed by the fact that speech, for example, may be entirely lost although only one hemisphere of the brain has suffered injury.

3. *Eye Dominance. See* Master Eye.

4. *Mendelian Dominance.* The tendency of one character to mask or hide its opposite when both are present in the parents. Thus, for example, if one parent comes from a family who are without exception brown-eyed and the

other comes from a comparable blue-eyed family, all the children of the first generation will be brown-eyed and for this reason brown eye color is said to be dominant over blue, which is called a recessive character. The tendency to blue eyes is not entirely lost in such a situation since some of the brown-eyed children of the first generation are able to transmit blue eyes to their own offspring if they mate with other hybrid individuals like themselves, or if they choose blue-eyed mates.

DYNAMOMETER—As used herein, an instrument for testing the strength of the hand grip.

ECHOLALIA—Echo speech. A stage in the development of speech in the child when he repeats words said to him with no understanding of their meaning. It also is an occasional symptom in some cases of mental disease in adults.

ELECTROENCEPHALOGRAPH—An instrument for amplifying and recording the very weak electrical currents which occur in the brain.

ENGRAM—The physiological record of a previous stimulus left in the brain or other nerve centers.

ETIOLOGICAL—Causative. In medicine, pertaining to the cause of disease.

EYEDNESS—*See* Master Eye.

FOOTEDNESS—Consistent preferential use of either the right or left foot for such unilateral functions as kicking, hopping, starting upstairs, etc.

FUSION, BINOCULAR—The combination of the images produced by the two eyes into one sensory impression.

GALVANOMETER—An instrument for detecting or recording electrical currents.

GENETICS—The study of heredity. Experimental genetics

has become a highly specialized field of biology in which the laws of heredity are studied by controlled matings of animals and plants.

GRAPHIC LANGUAGE—The use of drawn or written symbols to record or transmit ideas.

GYRUS (pl. Gyri)—The surface of the brain in all the higher mammals, including man, is marked by an intricate pattern of flat-topped ridges called *gyri* or *convolutions,* which are separated by narrow clefts called *sulci.* Angular gyrus—the brain cortex surrounding the end of the first temporal sulcus. It is the "critical area" for reading and is shown at 1 in Figure 3.

HANDEDNESS—*See* Master Hand.

HEMIANOPSIA—Blindness for one half the field of vision.

HEMIPLEGIA—Paralysis of one side of the body.

HEMISPHERE, CEREBRAL—Either lateral half of the brain.

HEREDITY—1. *Mendelian*—Following the laws of heredity as described by Mendel. *See* under Dominance.
2. *Sex-Linked*—A character or hereditary disease or defect which is transmitted consistently to children of one or the other sex only. The most commonly quoted disorders of this nature are *hemophilia* and *color blindness,* which are transmitted by unaffected mothers to their sons.
3. *Sex-Influenced*—A less rigid transmission to one sex than the *sex-linked.*
4. *Hereditary Lading*—The degree of taint or tendency toward the transmission of a disease or defect.

HOMOZYGOUS—Having exactly the same heredity. The nearest approach to this condition in experimental genetics is produced by many generations of very close inbreeding of animals or plants.

HYPERKINESIS—Overactivity or excessive movement.

Glossary

INFANTILISMS, SPEECH—Persistent childish defects in speech. Of these the lisp, the substitution of *w* for *r* and of *f* or *v* for *th* are common.

INTELLIGENCE QUOTIENT (I.Q.)—The ratio between an individual's mental age and his chronological age (*q.v.*).

INTERGRADES—1. *Genetic*—Various degrees of intermingling of hereditary characters.
    2. *Motor* (as used herein)—Intermixtures of right- and left-sidedness, as, for example, an individual who is right-handed and left-eyed, or one who performs some skilled acts with the left hand and others with the right.

KINAESTHESIS—Sensations from the muscles, tendons and joints by which muscular motion, weight, position, etc., are perceived. It is also from these sensations that new patterns of movement are in large part established.

LABIAL (As applied to speech)—Sounds in which movements or position of the lips play a part, such as *p, b, m*.

LATERAL (As applied to the brain)—The outer or convex surface of either hemisphere.

LESION, BRAIN—Damage to the structure of any part of the brain from injury or disease.

LINGUAL (As applied to speech)—Sounds which are formed with the aid of the tongue, such as *t, d*.

LINKAGES—*See* Association.

LOBE—One of the major anatomical subdivisions of the brain. The five lobes are indicated in Figure 1.

LOCALIZATION—*See* Cerebral Localization.

MASTER EYE—The eye which is habitually used for sighting.

MASTER HAND—The hand which is used by preference in skilled acts.

MASTER HEMISPHERE—The dominant half of the brain. *See* Dominance (2).

MEMORY—1. *Recognition memory* is that degree of familiarity with a given stimulus which permits its recognition when exposed again.

2. *Recall memory* is the somewhat greater degree of familiarity which permits the reviving of a stimulus in memory without renewed exposure.

MESIAL (As applied to the brain)—The inner or flat surface where the two hemispheres of the brain come together.

MNEMONIC—Pertaining to memory.

MOTOR AREA—*See* Area.

MOTOR NERVE CELLS—The large nerve cells in the spinal cord from which fibers run to the muscles and which directly control muscular movements. Also the giant nerve cells of the motor cortex in the brain which direct the activity of the spinal motor cells in voluntary movement.

MOTOR OVERFLOW—The term used in this volume to include involuntary movements of muscles, other than those directly concerned, during the spasms of stuttering and stammering. Some of the facial grimaces of many stutterers fall into this group.

MUSCLES, EXTRAOCULAR—The muscles on the outside of the eyeball which serve to turn it in its socket, as contrasted with the *intraocular* muscles whose duty is that of focusing the lens and changing the size of the pupil.

MYELIN (Myelin Sheaths)—The fat-like substance which forms an insulating sheath around the nerve fiber.

NEGATIVISM—A propensity to do the opposite of that which is requested.

NEOGRAPHISMS—The graphic equivalent of *neologisms* (*q.v.*).

Glossary

NEOLOGISMS—The invention of new words and particularly the use of word sounds in meaningless new combinations.

ONTOGENETIC—Origin and development of the individual, and thus to be contrasted with *phylogenetic* which is the evolution or ancestral history of a race or group of animals.

PATHOLOGICAL—Abnormal or diseased.

PARAGRAMMATISM—The type of errors seen in some cases of aphasia, characterized by confusion in the use and order of words and grammatical forms. *cf.* Agrammatism.

PARAPHASIA—The use of wrong words to express meaning as seen in some aphasics.

PHONETIC—Of or pertaining to speech sounds and their relation to graphic symbols.
  1. *Phonetic Synthesis*—The building up of a word from its phonetic units.
  2. *Phonetic Analysis*—The dissection of a spoken word into its component sounds.

PHYLOGENETIC—*See* Ontogenetic.

PHYLUM—One of the primary or main divisions of the animal or vegetable kingdoms.

PROPOSITIONAL SPEECH—Purposeful expression as contrasted with repetition of memorized material.

RECESSIVE HEREDITARY CHARACTER—*See* Dominance—Mendelian.

REVERSALS (As used in this volume)—1. *Kinetic*—Confusion or misreading a series of letters or words in which a progressional element enters, as when a whole word is read backward.
  2. *Static*—Confusion or mistakes in recognition of single letters which are alike except for their orientation, such as *b* and *d*.

SECLUSIVENESS—The tendency to withdraw from social contacts.
SEX-INFLUENCED—*See* Heredity.
SEX-LINKED—*See* Heredity.
SINISTRAD—To or toward the left.
SINISTRAL—Left. Also used as an abbreviation for a left-handed person.
SPASM—A sudden involuntary contraction of a muscle.
  1. *Clonic Spasm*—When characterized by alternating contraction and relaxation.
  2. *Tonic Spasm*—When persistent in contraction.
SPEECH MECHANISM—This consists of two parts, the *peripheral* and the *central*.
  1. The *peripheral* mechanism is made up of the lips, tongue, glottis, larynx, breathing apparatus and all of the nerves controlling these parts.
  2. The *central mechanism* is not so thoroughly understood but requires the collaboration of a number of areas in the cerebral cortex, notably those devoted to hearing and Broca's area, which is the brain center for motor control of speech.
STEREOPSIS (Stereoscopic Vision)—Perception of the third dimension in objects so that they appear as solid instead of as flat pictures.
STREPHOSYMBOLIA—A delay or difficulty in learning to read which is out of harmony with a child's general intellectual ability. At the outset it is characterized by confusion between similarly formed but oppositely oriented letters, and a tendency to a changing order of direction in reading.
SUSPENOPSIA—A tendency for the image arising in either eye to be entirely disregarded for a short period of time so that the individual is using one eye only for the time being.
SYNDROME—A complex of symptoms; a group of symptoms which occur together.

Glossary

THERAPY (a. Therapeutic)—The treatment of disease.
TIMBRE—The quality of a tone or sound.
TONIC—*See* Spasm.

UNILATERAL CEREBRAL DOMINANCE—*See* Dominance.

VIBRATO—Slight variations in pitch, less striking than the tremulo, which characterize emotional expression in speech and in singing.
VISUO-MOTOR CO-ORDINATION—The accurate adjustment of movement to accord with the incoming visual stimuli.

WORD-BLINDNESS—*See* Blindness.
WORD-DEAFNESS—*See* Deafness.

Index

Abnormal clumsiness. *See* Apraxia, developmental
Academic achievement
    developmental agraphia and, 99-100
    developmental alexia and, 90-99
    and emotional problems due to language disorder, 132, 133-36, 137
    mixed syndromes and, 126-27
    spelling problems and, 166
    treatment and, program for, 172-73, 277-78
Age
    chronological/mental, educational profile and, 74
    language acquisition and, 19–20, 64
    stuttering and, 124, 140, 194, 199
    teaching of writing and child's, 20
Agnosia, auditory, 29
Agrammatism, 95
    motor aphasia and, 47
Agraphia. *See also* Writing developmental (writing disability)
    academic achievement and, 99-100
    brain damage and, 110
    handedness and, 101–105, 110
    letters and, 99, 100, 104–105
    mirror writing and, 104–109
    purity of syndrome, 110
    treatment for, 179–85
    types of, 99–101
    vision-averted writing and, 109
    motor, defined, 44–45
Alexia (word blindness), 42, 45. *See also* Word blindness
    acquired, 152
    defined, 37–39
    developmental (reading disability)
    adademic achievement and, 90–99
    analyzed, 145–46
    arithmetic and 83–84, 171
    auditory development and, 74–77
    characteristic forms of, 72
    early investigations of, 69-72
    early uncorrected, 96-97
    graded series of, 72
    higher education and, 97–98
    intelligence and, 72–74, 95, 96
    laterality and, 90
    letter reversals and, 78–83, 93
    mirrored print and, 82–83
    numerical reversals and, 83–84, 171
    preventive program and, 176
    purity of syndromes in, compared with brain damage, 98–99, 110
    reading comprehension and, 73
    reading for a pastime and, 95–96
    residual, 92, 97
    as a sensory disorder, 90
    spelling and, 84–89, 93, 94, 95, 97, 98
    symptom, 73–74
    treatment for, 158–79
    vision and, 77–78
    vocabulary and, 92, 96
    writing and, 85, 89, 94, 95, 97
    speech sound reversals and, 146–48
Alphabetical letters. *See also* Sequencing (letters/sounds)
    alexia and, 37, 38
    alexia treatment and, 159–62
    developmental agraphia and, 99, 100, 104–105
    motor agraphia and, 45, 46
    phonetic cards for, 170
    reversals of, developmental alexia and, 78–83, 93, 94, 95, 97, 98, 145, 146
    reversals of, and stuttering, 196
    spelling, developmental alexia and, 71, 84–89, 93, 94, 95, 97, 98
Ambidexterity. *See* Handedness
Amnesia, 35
Amphiocularity, 52–53, 61, 121, 190
Analysis, phonetic. *See* Phonetic dissection
Anatomical studies, brain studies and, 25
Angular gyrus
    agensis in, 70

Angular gyrus *(continued)*
  alexia and, 39
  apraxia and, 47–48
  developmental alexia and, 70–71
  language disorders and damage to, 26
  maturity of, academic training of children and, 20
Animal experiments, the brain and, 23–34
Animal "language," 14. *See also* Language.
Animals
  brain size of, 30–31
  lack of unilateral cerebral dominance in, 27–28
Aniseikonia, 77
Aphasia, 25. *See also names of particular kinds of aphasia*
  acquired, 144
  auditory testing and, 41
  defined, 35–36
  sensory, 41
  word recognition and, 43–44
Apraxia, 105, 127, 146
  defined, 47–48
  delayed speech in, 190
  developmental (abnormal clumsiness), 120–22
  emotional problems and, 139
  interpretation of, 148–49
  treatment for, 190–94
  writing problems, and, 183
Area striata, 33
Arithmetic, 83–84, 171
Arteries, blocking of, brain damage and, 21–22
Attention span, teaching and, 170
Audiometer tests, word deafness and, 112, 114
Auditory agnosia, 29
Auditory aphasia (word deafness). *See also* Word deafness
  defined, 39–44
  speech sounds reversals and, 146–48
Auditory development. *See* Hearing
Ayres Handwriting Scale, 74, 101

Ballard, handedness and, 53
Behavior patterns, language delay/disorders and, 131–41
Birth paralysis, 48
Blending (phonetic). *See* Phonetic blending
Blindness. *See also* Alexia (word blindness); Word blindness
  congenital
    handedness and, 53–54
    word comprehension and, 25
  cortical, 29–30, 34
  mind, 29–30, 34
  peripheral, 28–29
Brain. *See also* Brain cortex; Brain damage; Cerebral dominance; Cerebral hemi-spheres; names of specific brain areas
  alexia and, 39
  animal experiments and, 23–24
  apraxia and, 47–48, 149
  auditory aphasia and, 43
  critical language areas of, 40 (figure)
  development of, language acquisition and, 16–17
  developmental alexia and, 70–71, 98
  emotional expression and, 15
  explanation of language disorder to children and, 199
  eyedness and, 54
  function of lobes in, 31, 32 (figure)
  language areas of, 40 (figure)
  laterality and, 48, 66–67
  mirror images and, 151–52
  motor agraphia and, 44, 45
  motor aphasia and, 47
  myelin in fibers of, 34
  physiological pattern in, 13–14, 143
  reading and, 152–53
  size of, in man and monkey, 30–31
  size of hemispheres of, 155–56
  studies of, 25
  vision and, 23–24, 28–29, 30, 31, 33–34, 35, 154–55
Brain cortex. *See also* Blindness, cortical; Brain; Deafness, cortical
  in animals/man, 23
  language understanding and, 36
  lesions of, language and, 143
  maturation of, 34
  motion and damage to, 28
  motor cells and, 153
  nerve cells/fibers of, 33
  vision and, 24
Brain damage. *See also* Brain; Brain cortex
  apraxia and, 121
  auditory aphasia and, 39
  blocking of artery in, 21–22
  developmental agraphia and, 110

developmental alexia and, 70–71
handedness and, 50–51
language disorder over-lapping and, 144
laterality and, 48
location of, language disorders and, 26
mind blindness/mind deafness and, 29–30
mixed syndromes and, 126
motor language losses and, 43–44
study of, language and, 21
stuttering and, 125
tumors and, 22–23
Broca's area, motor aphasia and, 47

Cannon, emotional expression experiments and, 15
Causation, language function disorders, 34–35, 72–73, 98–99, 133, 143, 199, 200
Cerebral dominance. *See also* Brain; Cerebral hemispheres
alexia and, 37,39
apraxia and, 121
auditory aphasia and, 39
brain structure and, 155
developmental alexia and, 70, 71
handedness and, 48–49, 50
handedness/language disorder and, 130
language disorders and, 27–35, 47
laterality and, 48, 142
stuttering and, 195
unilateral, 27–35, 51, 200
Cerebral hemispheres. *See also* Brain; Cerebral dominance
alexia and, 37, 39
aphasia and, 43
auditory aphasia and, 39
brain size and, 156
engram and, 152–55
functional superiority/structural superiority and, 156
language and, 68, 152
laterality, 48, 66–67, 142
physiological pattern in brain and, 13–14
Children. *See also* Infants; Testing
agraphic, treatment for, 179–85
alexic, treatment for, 158–79
aphasia and, 36
apraxia and, 120–22
apraxic, treatment of, 190–94
attention span of, teaching and, 170

behavorial/emotional problems in, with language disorders, 131–41
developmental agraphia and, 99–110
developmental alexia and, 69–99
developmental handedness histories and, 55–58
explaining language disorders to, 199
family ambitions for, language handicap and, 131–32
hemispheric dominance and, 48
hereditary factors/language disorders and, 127–30
individualized programs for teaching of, 170–72, 174–75
laterality studies of, 51–61
maternal overprotection of handicapped, 137–38
mixed syndromes in, 126–27
morale of, teaching and, 169
motor aphasic, treatment for, 187–90
motor intergrading of, 61–67
motor speech delay and, 118–20
stuttering/stammering and, 122–25
stuttering in, treatment for, 194–200
teaching reading and writing to, age consideration, 20
verbal language acquisition and, 16–20
word deaf, treatment for, 185–87
word deafness and, 111–18
Chorea, 123
Clincians, brain studies and, 25
Clumsiness. *See* Apraxia, developmental
Communication
animals and, 14
man and, 13
man's feeling tones and, 14
of meaning, 16
sign language and, 17
symbolic language and, 15
Compensations, reading disability and, 135, 139
Concepts, acquisition of, 114–15
Congenital, as a term, 69, 71
Consonant sounds
motor speech delay and, 119
speech development and, 17
Copying words, 71, 78, 88 (figure), 89 (figure), 184–85
Cortex, brain. *See* Brain cortex

Cortex, sensory, See Sensory cortices
Cortical blindness. See Blindness, cortical
Cortical deafness. See Deafness, cortical
Cortical defects, agenetic, 66

Deafness. See also Auditory aphasia (word deafness); Hearing; Word deafness
   congenital, word comprehension and, 25
   cortical, 29–30
   high frequency, 112–13, 114, 115 (figure), 137
   mind, 29–30
   organic, auditory aphasia and, 42
   reading and, 72
   regional, 113, 115 (figure), 186
   word deafness and, 112–13, 114
Dementia
   emotional expression and, 15
   word deafness and, 42
Developmental agraphia. See Agraphia, developmental
Developmental alexia. See Alexia, developmental
Developmental apraxia. See Apraxia, developmental
Developmental history, handedness and, 55–58
Developmental motor aphasia. See Motor aphasia, developmental
Developmental word deafness. See Word deafness, developmental
Dominance. See Cerebral dominance
Dysgraphia. See Agraphia, developmental
Dyslexia. See Alexia, developmental
Dyspraxia. See Apraxia, developmental
Dysphasia. See Aphasia

Echo Speech, 19. See also Speech
   auditory aphasia and, 41–42
   language acquisition and, 17–18
   motor aphasia and, 187, 188
   motor speech delay and, 119, 148
   word blindness/word deafness and, 116, 147
Education. See Academic achievement
Educational profile
   developmental agraphia and, 100 (figure)
   developmental alexia and, 74, 75 (figure), 76 (figure), 86 (figure)
Elision of engrams, 152–55

Emotion. See also Emotional problems
   animal "language" and, 14
   expression of, and motor aphasia, 46
   language acquisition and, 16, 18–19
   man's, communication of, 14–15
Emotional problems. See also Emotion
   developmental alexia and, 72
   from frustration in motor speech delay, 120
   language delay/disorders and, 131–41, 157, 168, 199
   stuttering and, 199
Engram, elision of and developmental alexia, 152–55
Enunication
   clear, and aphasic patients, 42
   in teaching the motor aphasic, 188
   in teaching spelling, 166, 167
   in teaching the word deaf, 186
Environmental influences
   on emotional problems in language disorder children, 131–32
   in language acquisition, 19
Examinations. See Tests Eyedness, 48. See also Laterality; Vision
   motor aphasic treatment and, 189
   motor intergrading and, 61, 62
   studies of, 51–55
   and teaching alexic patients, 174

Face, paralysis of, motor aphasia and, 45
Familial occurrence of language disorders, 90. See also Heredity
Feeblemindedness, word deafness and, 115–16, 138
Finger pointing, teaching alexics and, 164
Flash-card method and teaching of reading, 158, 175
Flechsig's studies of brain development (myelinization), 34
Footedness, 48, 55. See also Laterality
Frontal lobe, 31, 32 (figure)

Galen, "ambilevous" children and, 120
Galvanometer testing for handedness, 59–60. See also Testing
Golla, handedness and, 59–60
Gould, eyedness and, 53, 54
Graphic spelling. See Spelling, graphic
Gyri. See Angular gyrus; Precentral gyrus; Temporal gyri

Handedness. *See also* Laterality; Left-handedness
  agraphia treatment and, 179–85
  ambidexterity and, 65–66, 130
  brain damage and, 50–51
  cerebral dominance and, 48–49, 155–56
  change in, 50–51
  developmental agraphia and, 101–105, 110
  developmental alexia and, 90
  developmental history and, 55–58
  eyedness and, 52, 53, 54
  hereditary, 128–30, 155–56
  hereditary right, 49
  language disorders and hereditary factors, 127–30
  motor aphasics treatment and, 189, 190
  motor speech delay and, 119
  retraining and, 90
  sidedness and, motor intergrading, 61–67
  studies of, 55–61, 62
  stuttering and, 60, 124, 125, 194–95, 196
  teaching alexics and, 173–74
  testing for, 58–61
  training and, 49, 50, 51, 56–57, 59
  word deafness and, 118
Handwriting. *See* Writing
Hearing
  cerebral dominance and, 29–30
  development of, developmental alexia and, 74–77
  sensory aphasia and, 41
  and vision and word comprehension, 25
  word deafness and, 111, 113, 147
Hemianopsia, 29, 37
Hemispheres, cerebral. *See* Cerebral hemispheres
Heredity
  family patterns, of, 129 (figure)
  handedness and, 48–49, 127–30, 155–56
  language acquisition and, 69
  language disability and, 127–30, 155–56, 200
  motor intergrading and, 62, 63, 66
  stuttering and, 195
High blood pressure, speech/reading disturbances and, 22
High frequency deafness. *See* Deafness, high frequency
Hinshelwood, developmental alexia and, 69–70, 71
History, developmental. *See* Developmental history
Hyperkinesis, stuttering and, 140. *See also* Overactivity

Infantile paralysis and handedness, 51
Infantilisms (speech), 120
Infants. *See also* Children
  animal "language" and, 14, 15
  babbling and, 17
  brain cortex and, 34
  eyedness and, 53
  laterality and, 48
Intelligence
  development of, language disorder influence on, 133, 135
  developmental alexia and, 72–74, 95, 96
  explaining disorder to children and, 199
  reading comprehension and, 73
  word deafness and, 114–15
Iowa Psychopathic Hospital, 60
  reading study, 83, 157
  teaching methods and, 175

Jargon aphasia, 41, 199

Kinesthesis, 28, 31, 127, 148, 159
  producing letters and, 162, 183
Kleist
  paragrammatism and, 43
  "sentence muteness" and, 47, 178

Laboratory investigations, brain studies and, 25
Lalognosis, 18
Language. *See also* Language disorders
  alexia and, 39
  animal, 14
  brain areas and, 40 (figure)
  brain size and, 31
  child's acquisition of verbal, 16–20
  development, critical periods of, 62
  faculty, functions of, 157
  foreign, developmental alexia and, 94, 97
  graphic, stuttering and, 124
  handedness and development of, 62, 64
  loss and brain control, 66–67
  motor, losses, 43–44
  motor patterns and development of, 68–69

Language *(continued)*
  sign, Paget's thesis of, 16–17
  symbolic, 15, 16–17, 18, 19
Language disorders. *See also* Language; *name of specific disorder*
  apraxia and, 121
  ambidexterity and, 130
  brain damage and, 21, 22, 26
  brain studies and, 25–26
  cerebral dominance and, 27–35
  developmental delay and, 143–44
  emotional problems caused by, 131–41, 157, 168, 199
  explaining to child/parent, 199–200
  expressive, 95
  familial occurrence, of, 90
  handedness and, 90, 101–105, 110, 118, 125, 127–30, 189–90, 194–95, 196
  heredity and, 127–30
  interpretation of, 144–56
  memory and, 144
  motor aphasia and, 45–47
  neurological interpretation of, 143
  overlapping of, 144–45
  physiological nature of, 143
Language Research Project of the New York Neurological Institute, 41, 60, 110, 157
Lashley, brain damage thesis of, 26
Laterality, 142. *See also* Eyedness; Footedness; Handedness
  developmental alexia and, 90
  general overview of, 48–51
  language disorders and hereditary, 127–28
  studies in, 51–61
Left-handedness. *See also* Handedness
  agraphia treatment and, 179–83
  double, 120, 190
  enforced right-handedness and, 50, 51
  familial, 90
  hereditary, 48
  hereditary factors and language disorders and, 127–30
  "masked", 101
  motor speech delay and, 119
  prejudice against, 49–50, 56–57
  stuttering and, 125, 194–95, 196
  training to right-sidedness and, 64, 105
Letters, alphabetical. *See* Alphabetical letters
Limbic lobe, 31, 32 (figure)
Lip reading, 113

Manoptoscope, testing eyedness and, 53. *See also* Testing
Manual dexterity, 13
  apraxia and, 47
  developmental alexia and, 90
  unilateral, 27
Marie, Pierre, 48, 70
Master hand, paralysis of, motor aphasia and, 45. *See also* Handedness
Memory
  reading disability and, 145
  sense of direction and, 78
  sequencing and, 147
  teaching methods and, 173
  word deaf treatment and, 187
  word comprehension and, 18
  of words
    angular gyrus and, 26, 70
    developmental alexia and, 71, 84, 85
Mind blindness. *See* Blindness, mind
Mind deafness. *See* Deafness, mind
Mirrored print, 82–83
Mirror reading, 150, 151–52, 82
Mirror writing, 104–109, 151, 184
Morale of child, teaching and, 169
Morgan, developmental alexia and, 69
Motion, motor cortex and, 24, 28
Motor agraphia. *See* Agraphia, motor
Motor aphasia
  defined, 45–47
  developmental (motor speech delay), 118–20
  sequencing and, 148
  treatment for, 187–90
Motor cortex (brain), motion and, 24, 28
Motor intergrading
  defined, 49
  developmental alexia and, 90
  motor asphasics treatment and, 189
  studies of, 61–67
  stuttering and, 125, 195
Motor language losses, 43–44. *See also* Motor aphasia
Motor nerve cells, 153
Motor patterns
  apraxia and, 121, 192
  developmental alexia and, 90
  difficulty in learning, apraxia and, 121–22
  handedness and, 58

language development and, 68–69
sidedness and, 61, 62, 66
stuttering and, 194
Motor speech apparatus
auditory aphasia and, 42
stuttering and, 123–24
Motor speech delay. *See* Motor aphasia, developmental
Motor unrest. *See* Hyperkinesis; Overactivity
Muscles, stuttering and contraction of, 123
Muteness, "sentence," 47, 178
Mutism, 119
Myelin, 34

Negativism of child, 136–37
Neographisms, 39, 87, 88 (figure)
word deafness and, 117, 147
Nervous system, 13
animal "language" and, 15
bilateral symmetry of, 14
Neurological explanation of language disorders, 150
New York Neurological Institute, Language Reserach Project of, 41, 60, 110, 157
Nonsense material, word recognition and, 80, 91, 163
Nouns in speech development, 19
Numerical reversals, 83–84, 171. *See also* Sequencing

Occipital lobe, 31, 32 (figure)
Occipital pole, 33, 54
Optic thalami, 23–24
Oral reading. *See* Reading, oral
Oral spelling. *See* Spelling, oral
Order of recall, writing. *See* Sequencing
Orientation, spatial, 78
Overactivity, 170. *See also* Hyperkinesis
in stuttering, 140
in word deafness, 116

Paget, Richard, sign language thesis and, 16–17
Paragrammatism, 43
Parietal lobe, 31, 32 (figure)
apraxia and, 47–48
Parson, handedness/eyedness and, 52, 53, 54
"Pencil facilitation," teaching stutterers and, 197–98

Peripheral blindness. *See* Blindness, peripheral
Phonetic blending
motor aphasia treatment and, 187–88
motor speech delay and, 148
sequencing and, 162
Phonetic dissection
as guide to spelling, 165–67, 170, 175–76
stuttering and, 195–96
word deafness treatment and, 185–87, 188
Physiological record. *See* Engram
Precentral gyrus, motor agraphia and, 45
Profanity, motor aphasia and, 46
Propositional speech, 198, 199. *See also* Speech

Reading. *See also* Alexia, developmental
alexia and, 38, 39
brain damage and, 21, 22, 26
causes of failure in, 72
cerebral dominance and, 27 28
discovering disability in, 176–77
emotional disturbance and handicap in, 132–36
errors, 79, 91–92
finger-pointing method of teaching, 164
flash-card teaching and, 158, 175
grammatical sequence and, 93
handedness and, hereditary factors, 128
language disorder overlapping and, 144–45
lip, 113
loss of, and speech, 24
narrative, and teaching of, 168–69
oral, 98, 185
capacity for, developmental alexia and, 87
high standards of, accuracy and, 169
reading and, 92–93
retraining program and, 172, 173, 179
spelling and, 97, 172–73
stuttering and, 197
as pastime, 95–96
selective loss of, retardation in, 34–35
sentence length and, 92
silent, 91, 97, 172

Reading (continued)
   simple vocabulary as teaching problem for, 169
   spelling problems and, 164–68
   stuttering and, 124, 125, 126, 197
   teaching of, child's age and, 20
   teaching of, related to disability, 175
   trace-sounding method of teaching, 159–62
   word deafness and confusion in, 116
Reading disability. See Alexia, developmental; Strephosymbolia
Regional deafness. See Deafness, regional
Research data, sources of, 157
Residual strephosymbolia, 92, 96–97
Retraining. See also Training; Treatment
   alexia and, 38
   emotional considerations and, 131, 135, 137
Reversals. See Alphabetical letters; Sequencing; Spelling
Right-handedness. See Handedness; Left-handedness
Rockefeller Foundation, 157

St. Vitus' dance, 123
School examinations. See Tests
School work. See Academic achievement
Seclusiveness
   apraxia and, 139
   motor speech delay and, 139
   word deafness and, 138
Senses, brain hemispheres and, 28, 31
Sensory aphasia, 41, 43, 46, 116
Sensory cortices, handedness patterns and, 173
Sensory disorder, 90
Sensory functions, levels of, 31–33
"Sentence muteness," 47, 178
Sentences
   length of, reading disability and, 92
   speech development and, 19
   word deafness and, 116
Sequencing (letter/sounds). See also Alphabetical letters, reversals of; Numerical reversals; Sound(s)
   alexia treatment and, 162–64
   importance of, 158
   language acquisition and, 19
   language disorder overlapping and, 145, 150
   letter sounds/stuttering and, 149
   memory for, 145
   motor speech delay and, 148
   reading disability and, 145–46
   spelling (order of recall), 71, 85
   word blindness/word deafness and, 146–48
   word deafness treatment and, 185
   writing disability and, 146, 184
Sherrington, flicker experiments of, 29
Sidedness. See Eyedness; Footedness; Handedness; Laterality; Motor intergrading
Sign language, 16–17, 119. See also Language
Sound(s). See also Phonetic blending; Phonetic dissection; Sequencing (letters/sounds)
   child's speech development and, 17–18
   confusing similarities of, and developmental alexia, 91–92
   developmental alexia and, 74, 93
   letter association and, 89
   trace-sound method of teaching, 159–62
   understanding of aphasia and, 41
   word deafness and, 112, 113
Spasms, stuttering and, muscular, 123
Specific reading disability.
   See Alexia, developmental
speech, 13. See also Aphasia; Motor aphasia; Propositional speech
   apraxia and, 121–22
   birth paralysis and disorders in, 48
   brain damage and, 21, 26
   cerebral dominance and, 27, 28
   concept acquisition and, 114–15
   confusion in, word deafness and, 116–17
   development of, in child, 17–20
   developmental motor aphasia and, 118–20
   disturbances in, high blood pressure and, 22
   echo, 17–18, 19, 41–42, 116, 119, 147, 148, 187, 188
   handedness injury and, 65
   hemispheric dominance and, 48
   language acquisition and, 16–17
   language disorder overlapping and, 144–45
   loss of, reading and, 24
   motor agraphia and, 44

sensory aphasia and, 41
slow delivery of, and aphasic patients, 42
spelling and accuracy of, 167
stuttering and, 122–25, 126
training, motor aphasics and, 187–90
word deafness and, 111–13, 116–18
Spelling. *See also* Alphabetical letters; Sequencing (letters/sounds)
  alexia and, 39
  apraxia and, 47
  auditory discrimination and, 165–66
  developmental alexia and, 71, 84–89, 93, 94, 95, 97, 98, 145–46
  association with, 164
  letter reversals and, 78–83, 93
  treatment and, 164–68
  emotional problems and handicap in, 133, 134
  graphic, 45, 94, 95, 165, 166, 167
  language disorder overlapping and, 144–45
  motor agraphia and, 44
  oral, 45, 85, 165, 166
  oral reading and, 93, 97, 172–73
  phonetic dissection as guide to learning, 165–67, 170, 175–76
  stuttering and, 126
  visual recall and, 93
  word deafness treatment and, 187
Spinal cord, 153
Stanford-Binet examination, 74
Strephosymbolia. *See also* Alexia, developmental
  developmental alexia as, 69
  defined, 71
Stroke, language faculty and, 22
Stuttering, 142
  charactertistics of, 122–25
  emotional problems, and, 139–41
  handedness and, 60, 124, 125, 194–95, 196
  hereditary factors and, 128, 130
  home discipline and, 198–99
  hyperkinesis and, 140
  left-handedness and, 125, 194–95, 196
  mixed syndromes and, 126
  motor speech delay and, 120
  "pencil facilitation" and, 197–98
  treatment for, 194–200
Symbolic language, 15, 16–17. *See also* Language

echoing and, 18
emotional expression in children and, 19

Teaching. *See* Reading, Retraining; Training; Treatment; Writing
Temper tantrums
  motor speech delay and, 139
  stuttering and, 140
  word deafness and, 137
Temporal gyri (second and third), auditory aphasia and, 43
Temporal lobe, 31, 32 (figure)
Testing. *See also* Tests
  apraxics, 121
  auditory, aphasia and, 41
  eyedness, 52–53
  handedness, 58–61, 62
  hearing for word deafness, 111, 112, 114
  intelligence, and developmental alexia, 73, 74
  laterality, 51
  motor, handedness/stuttering and, 194
  writing skills, 182–83
Tests. *See also* Testing
  failures on, writing disability and, 136
  understanding of, by alexic children, 84, 91, 93, 95, 96, 97
Therapy. *See* Retraining; Training; Treatment
Trace-sound method of teaching, 159–62
Training. *See also* Retraining; Treatment
  academic, child's age and, 20
  apraxics, 191–92
  auditory, developmental alexia and, 77
  handedness and, 49, 50, 51, 56–57, 59, 64, 65, 66
  methods of, language acquisition and, 19
  mixed syndromes and difficulty in, 126–27
  mutism and speech, 119
  reading and stuttering, 125
  word deaf children, 138
Travis, handedness and, 60
Treatment. *See also* Retraining; Training
  of aphasic patients, tutor's speech delivery/enunciation and, 42–43

Treatment *(continued)*
 apraxia, 190–94
 associative linkages and, 164
 college students, 177–78
 developmental agraphia, 179–85
 developmental alexia, 158–79
 duration, 171
 education of tutors for, 178–79
 experiments in, 156–57
 explaining disorder to child/parent and, 199–200
 first steps toward, 157–58
 individualized programs for, 170–72, 174–75
 mistrained left-handers, 179–83
 motor aphasia, 187–90
 oral reading, 172–73
 older students, 172–73
 principles of teaching, 158
 sensory reinforcement and, 159
 sequencing and, importance of, 158
 stuttering, 194–200
 timing of sessions, 171
 word deafness, 185–87
Tumors, brain damage and, 22–23

Verbs
 in speech development, 19
 word deafness and, 117
Vision, 13. *See also* Blindness; Eyedness
 alexia and, 37
 brain structure and, 23–24, 154–55
 cerebral dominance and, 28–29, 30, 31, 33–34, 35
 developmental agraphia and, 109
 developmental alexia and, 77–78
 developmental apraxia and, 121
 hearing and, in word comprehension, 25
 sequencing and, 147–48
 visuo-motor coordination and, 78
Vocabulary
 auditory, developmental alexia and, 77
 developmental alexia and, 92, 96
 of normal child, 19–20
 reading errors and, 91–92
 reading/speech loss and, 24
 teaching of reading and, 169
 word deafness and, 116
Vowels. *See also* Vowel sounds
 motor speech delay and, 119
 phonetic blending and, 187–88
 word deafness and, 113

Vowel sounds. *See also* Vowels
 speech development and, 17
 teaching spelling and, 165

Wile, eyedness and, 53
Word blindness, 30, 34. *See also* Alexia (word blindness)
 congenital, 69, 71
Word deafness, 30, 126, 127. *See also* Auditory aphasia developmental
 concept acquisition and, 114–15
 confusion in speech and, 116–17, 118
 emotional problems and, 136–38
 hearing and, 111
 overactivity and, 116
 speech and, 111, 112, 113
 treatment for, 185–87
 true deafness and, 112–13
Words. *See also* Alexia; Auditory aphasia; Phonetic dissection; Word deafness
 comprehension of, speech and, 18
 memory of, angular gyrus and, 26
 motor aphasia and, 46–47
 nonsense, 80
 recognition of, aphasia and, 43–44
 developmental alexia and, 78
 sequences of, language acquisition and, 19
 used in commands to aphasic patients, 43
 vision/hearing and, 25
Writing. *See also* Agraphia
 alexia and, 38, 39
 apraxia and, 122
 brain damage and, 21, 26
 brain and development of, 17
 cerebral dominance and, 27, 28
 copying/dictation and, 78, 88 (figure), 89 (figure), 184–85
 developmental alexia and, 85, 87, 89, 94, 95, 97
 emotional disturbances and handicap in, 136
 handedness and, 60, 63
 motor agraphia and, 44–45
 motor aphasia and, 46
 and overlapping language disorders, 144–45, 150
 paper/hand position in, 181–82
 stuttering and, 124, 125, 126, 197
 teaching of, child's age and, 20
 treatment for disability in, 179–85
 typewriter use and, 47, 184